# SUFFERING IN SLOW MOTION

# Suffering in Slow Motion

*Help for a Long Journey Through Dementia
and Other Terminal Illnesses*

PAMALA KENNEDY
RICHARD KENNEDY

SERVANT PUBLICATIONS
ANN ARBOR, MICHIGAN

Vine Books is an imprint of Servant Publications especially designed to serve
evangelical Christians.

---

**Servant Publications—Mission Statement**

We are dedicated to publishing books that spread the gospel of Jesus
Christ, help Christians to live in accordance with that gospel, promote
renewal in the church, and bear witness to Christian unity.

---

Unless otherwise indicated, Scripture quotations used in this book are taken
from the Holy Bible, New International Version. Copyright 1973, 1978, 1984
International Bible Society. Used by permission of Zondervan Bible Publishers.
Scripture quotations marked (NLT) are taken from the *Holy Bible*, New Living
Translation, copyright 1996. Used by permission of Tyndale House Publishers,
Inc., Wheaton, Illinois 60189. All right reserved. Quotations marked THE
MESSAGE are from *The Message*, copyright by Eugene H. Peterson 1993, 1994,
1995. Used by permission of NavPress Publishing Group.

The personal anecdotes that appear in this book are true and have been freely
shared with the author and used by permission of the individuals involved.

Published by
Servant Publications
P.O. Box 8617
Ann Arbor, Michigan 48107
www.servantpub.com

Cover design: Steve Eames

03 04 05 06 10 9 8 7 6 5 4 3 2 1

Printed in the United States of America
ISBN 1-56955-359-9

*Library of Congress Cataloging-in-Publication Data*
Kennedy, Pamala Condit.
  Suffering in slow motion : help for a long journey through dementia
and other terminal illnesses / Pamala Kennedy, Richard Kennedy.
      p. cm.
Includes bibliographical references.
  ISBN 1-56955-359-9 (alk. paper)
  1. Church work with the terminally ill. 2. Terminal care–Religious
aspects. 3. Terminally ill–Religious life. I. Kennedy, Richard. II.
Title.
  BV4460.6.K43 2003
  248.8'61–dc21

                                                              2003012393

# CONTENTS

*Introduction*                                                    / 7

**Part I: When Trouble Comes Knocking**

  1. Life in the Cocoon                                 / 15
  2. What Will Become of Me?                            / 35
  3. What Is Suffering?                                 / 51
  4. Trading Fear for Trust                             / 63

**Part II: I Will Fear No Evil**

  5. Keys to Living With Loss                           / 83
  6. When God *Doesn't*                                 / 95
  7. Staying Close                                      / 109
  8. The God of All Comfort                             / 127

**Part III: Survival Skills**

  9. The Importance of Family and Friends               / 149
10. Making the Hard Decisions                                    / 157
11. Prayer and Journaling: Seeking the Father's Heart / 171
12. The Long View: Keeping Your Eyes on the Horizon / 185

In Summary                                                       / 201
Epilogue                                                         / 205
Appendix: *How and where to get help from home*                 / 209
Notes                                                            / 221

# INTRODUCTION

In our heart of hearts we knew that someday we would tell our story of *suffering in slow motion*. It's the story of our family's journey through discovering, denying, and then dealing with the terminal illness of one family member.

It's not every day you pick up a book about pain and suffering. If you chose this book by its title, it's a sure sign you are at a point of need in your life. Far from being just a personal testimonial of the trials our family has met and conquered, this book is meant to be a companion to all who are walking through their own journeys of suffering, illness or loss. In a culture awash in "how to" books, we call this a "must do" book. We say "must do" because people who suffer must do so against their wills. Tragedy is no respecter of persons. It comes as an intruder.

**Richard:** I had just received my Doctor of Ministry degree from Fuller Theological Seminary and had just assumed the senior pastor position at Los Gatos Christian Church in California. I said to my wife, Pamala, "Hon, God has been preparing us all of our lives for the ministry we are going to be doing for the next ten years!"

**Pamala:** It was those very words I reflected on during the drive home from the University of California Medical Center on October 9, 1997. My husband, Dr. Richard Kennedy, and I had been seeking a reason for the unexplainable physical, emotional and mental changes he had been experiencing for the past year. This day was the culmination of a three-month study to find out what was wrong with him, a seemingly healthy forty-seven-year-old man at the height of his career. The drive home was filled with tears and my thoughts were skyrocketing off in every direction. Questions remained unanswered. How long will Richard live? What can we expect? And the question I hated most—*Can I do this?* Can I live while watching Richard die?

Richard and I have been "can do" overachievers all of our lives. We've always taken on a new challenge like kids in a candy store—"Just let us at it!" But the news of a degenerative brain disease, one that has no treatment and no way of fighting back, was the worst sort of challenge. Were we to just sit back and wait while it took Richard from us?

Since we were kids, our names have been said together—Richard *and* Pamala. We met at church camp when I was fourteen and he was sixteen. To some it might appear that we have lived a charmed life. And as far as ministry goes that is true. We have pastored great churches and have traveled to many countries telling people about Jesus. Richard has earned four degrees, and I authored a book (before this one) that opened the doors to speaking opportunities as well as radio and television appearances across the country.

**Richard:** A part of me says I must know how to suffer perfectly in order to be qualified to write this book. But I can assure you, that is not the case. Like a baseball player I have run the bases of denial, anger, frustration and depression only to be left exhausted in mind, body and spirit.

This journey of suffering has truly been in *slow motion.* For some, death is instant, tragic and without advance warning or time to prepare. But for others the news of one's death is given long before the actual event. Months—or even years—of suffering can precede a person's death. The culprit may be cancer, Alzheimer's disease or Parkinson's disease, to mention only a few. They too are slow, steady, and just as deadly. Whatever the cause, it is with those who suffer in slow motion—and with their families and friends—that we want to share our story with the hope it will bring to you some source of courage and perseverance.

**Pamala:** If you and your family are dealing with a terminal illness, then there was a day when you got the news. You heard the doctor say the words, but you could never imagine the journey that lay just ahead of you. In the early stages of our ordeal, we found very little practical help as we scrambled to find our way. So now, with this book, our desire is to reach out to others who are facing the same pain. Our story is sad; someone has to die. But we are not in search of sympathy. Rather, we hope to offer those who suffer and those who care for someone who suffers a place where your feelings are validated, and where you might find comfort in knowing that others have traveled the road ahead of you.

The book is divided into three sections. The first section tells our story in detail and how our family has coped with this terminal illness. The second section attempts to answer the question, "Why?" In every case of suffering, this question is sure to arise. The final section deals with practical survival skills.

Since Richard and I are both writing this book, you will see our names in **boldface type** throughout, indicating who is writing a particular section. I would also like to explain that the majority of Richard's writing has been taken directly from his personal journal in which he wrote during the first two years of his illness. Keep in mind that Richard's illness is one that is psychotic in nature, so it has impaired his ability to think rationally and appropriately. However, he can also carry on intelligently at times, a contrast that was perfectly demonstrated in the movie, "A Beautiful Mind." This is one of the challenges the illness has presented to our family: We often hear people say, "He seems so normal." But as the years of the illness have worn on, his ability to function normally has slowly diminished.

Currently—five years into the illness—Richard must live in a completely controlled environment where he has no responsibilities whatsoever. He cannot survive without several medications, which he must take morning and night. Two years ago he began taking one of his medications, called Depakote, at a dosage of 500 milligrams per day; now his dosage has increased to 3500 milligrams per day. He takes five other controlled-substance medications and the dosages for those also have increased tremendously over the past five years. We are thankful for these medications because they have allowed Richard a better quality of life, but please do not equate this with a normal existence.

I felt it necessary to address this before you begin to read because you will be amazed at the beauty of Richard's writing throughout this book. I have taken the liberty to edit all of his writing for the sake of continuity and clarity.

*Even when I walk through the dark*
*valley of death, I will not be afraid, for*
*you are close beside me. Your rod and*
*your staff protect and comfort me.*

PSALM 23:4, NLT

Richard and Pamala Kennedy
Owasso, Oklahoma
2002

**Part I**

**WHEN TROUBLE COMES KNOCKING**

# ONE

## Life in the Cocoon

**Richard:** After being the picture of health for forty-six years, I was traveling in the Philippines with Pamala visiting missionaries our church supported. Upon our arrival I was anxious, cranky, irrational and downright obnoxious. I thought maybe it was mega-jet lag from the long trip. I was a terrible guest for the first few hours and Pamala finally talked me into taking two Tylenol PMs and going to bed. From that time on we referred to this behavior as an "episode."

### The "River of De-Nile"
**Pamala:** I stayed by myself to rest the next day while Richard and the two missionaries went to a small village on the outskirts of Manila. Richard and I had arrived the day before from Tokyo, so I knew he was desperately in need of some good rest too. But I was not prepared for what happened later that day.

I heard the car pull into the drive and the car door slam. Kathy, the missionary's wife, opened the door of the house and said, "Pamala, there is something terribly wrong with Pastor Richard. You need to go help him." The look on her face told me that whatever happened had frightened her. I went to help Richard then, and now, five years later, I am still helping him daily through the episodes that first became apparent on that trip.

When I opened the door and went outside to see what had happened to Richard, he was leaning against the outside wall of the porch. He was deathly white and mumbling over and over, "I have to get out of here; I have to get out of here." I spoke softly to him, while coaxing him into the house and into our bedroom. I tried talking with him, but he made no sense. He was angry, raising his voice, pushing me about and telling me to get him out of this place. I remained calm while explaining to him that we were far, far away from home, and that he must relax and lie down. Still, his agitation continued for the next three days. Needless to say, our missionary friends were confused and concerned. I did my best to excuse his behavior by saying he had been pushing himself too hard back home and he just needed some time off. They agreed, and reluctantly let it go at that.

After three days of solitude Richard was up and running again, full of energy and mentally sharp. He had almost no recollection of the previous three days; in fact, he insisted I was blowing it all out of proportion, and he was fine.

This type of behavior continued off and on for the next year. I could not figure out what caused it or when it would start. He would seem fine, and then suddenly change before my eyes. The changes were dramatic. He would become angry in an instant—upset over everything and anything, with no flexibility at all. He would get a lost look in his eyes. His hands would turn almost white, his arms would hang lifelessly at his side, and his shoulders would slump. He became confused, unable to make even the simplest of choices, like what to choose for lunch from a menu. He became verbally and physically abusive to me. Much of my frustration was that he had no memory of these episodes, and when I mentioned them, he denied them. I actually began to doubt myself.

Before long Richard's bizarre behavior began manifesting itself at work or when we were with friends. I received calls from his staff reporting he had done something out of character. Our friends began asking me if "things" were all right. One day, while we were on an outing with long-time friends, Richard had a full-blown episode. The man driving the car actually pulled over and told Richard to stop his bad behavior or get out of the car. Richard got out of the car. I was crying, trying to explain that something was wrong with him. Our friends knew only that Richard was acting like a jerk. After this I did not accept any invitations for social activities for us; Richard was too unpredictable. Thus my life of "protecting" him began.

### Guarding Richard

**Pamala:** I started keeping track of Richard's episodes, trying to figure out what would set them off, because until they began, Richard Kennedy was one of the most controlled, even-tempered, steady and kind persons I had ever met. After a few months of keeping track of things, and praying for wisdom, I could finally see a pattern forming. Richard's dramatic change was likely to occur:

- When he got overly tired or stressed
- When anything changed in his schedule
- When he was in a crowded place
- When more than one thing was going on, like TV and conversation

- When confined in a car or small room
- When things did not go his way
- When he felt rushed or we needed to hurry
- When subjected to movement of lights or people
- When faced with sudden noise or disruptions.

I set out to literally keep all of these things from happening to him on a daily basis—at home and at work. I began going to the office with him, even attending meetings, and asking his assistant to keep certain things from happening during his day. But in spite of our efforts, his episodes started getting worse and occurring more often. It became evident to friends and family that something was seriously wrong with Richard. It would be our trip to India that finally convinced Richard that he was very ill.

**Nightmare in India**
**Pamala:** The following year we took another trip to visit missionaries. The trip was a nightmare from beginning to end. Remember all of the events that would set off these episodes? Well there was no way to keep situations like these from happening while traveling in a third world country like India. The frustrations of travel provoked Richard into his worse episode we had seen. It was this behavior that would finally convince us there was something seriously wrong.

One evening after a full day of teaching and spending a long evening with the missionary couple, I could see that Richard had reached his saturation point and that we needed to get to our room immediately so he could rest. But he had already gotten too tired and was severely agitated. Once we were alone in our room he began to assault me physically. He held me down with his body, and forced my face into a pillow so I could not breathe or scream out for help. I felt I would not survive this attack, but I prayed for God's help and suddenly Richard came to "himself" and released his hold on me. There would be more times like this in the future—worse times, as a matter of fact—when I would feel that my life was at risk. But it was seeing the bruises from this incident the next day that first convinced Richard something was seriously wrong. By the time we made our way back to the United States, Richard was more than ready to find out what it was.

### Seeking Help

**Richard:** I began looking for answers with my family physician and using the referral system of our health maintenance organization (HMO). What a hassle! My compassion level for people dealing with health issues and working within the health "system" immediately skyrocketed. One of my great struggles that first year was knowing that something was wrong with me—but what? It was the source of great anxiety for me, like a constant wrestling match with my own mortality. On top of that was the frustration of feeling that I had to fight with my HMO to get the help I needed. As I'm sure you're aware, in an HMO, each individual has a primary care physician. Rarely is the primary care physician a specialist, so he or she must refer you to various specialists, but the HMO has to approve your visit before you can see the specialist. Often somebody sitting behind a desk declined my referrals— somebody I had never even had the opportunity to meet (and that was probably a good idea!). I can spell HMO another way: F-R-U-S-T-R-A-T-I-O-N. Many of you know exactly what I mean.

Fortunately, my secretary had worked in a physician's office and knew the ins and outs of how the process worked. She asked me to give her my files (which by now had become quite thick). She wrote appeal letters and documented my case. In the end I got every test, saw every specialist, and received every imaging scan I needed. Thank you, Robyn.

I was sent to Stanford Medical Center in Palo Alto, where I was scanned from head to foot in search of a tumor of some sort. The reports came back negative. But my episodes continued. My energy level was decreasing, even though I visited my health club three to four times a week. My moods ranged from anxiety to depression to anger and everything in between. Something was wrong.

## A Trip to the Shrink

**Richard:** Next on the schedule was a visit to a psychologist and a psychiatrist. Somehow I thought seeing a "shrink" was a less-than-manly thing to do. But I must admit it was there I first began to find some relief. The psychiatrist explained about how the brain functions and how various medications could help. Over the next few months, I felt like a laboratory rat. I went through a gamut of medications in attempt to find the right balance. But medications were not a substitute for a diagnosis. We wanted to know what we were dealing with.

Finally I was admitted as a patient at the Medical Center at the University of California at San Francisco (UCSF). I was patient #345-34-58-6. I still have my "blue card." They had a special Memory Clinic & Alzheimer's Center as a part of their Langley Porter Psychiatric Institute. Dr. James Mastrianni was the medical director of the clinic. He was cordial, professional, and among the best in the nation in his field of research. He introduced me to the medical team who would be working with Pamala and me over the next few months in an attempt to give us an accurate diagnosis. This is my journal entry from Thursday, August 28, 1997:

> I can't recap the past two to three months, but it has been up and down. It's one day of pain and tears, and a day or two to recover before the cycle begins again. My experiences at UCSF have been frightening at times, but I know (or at least I think) they are going to make an accurate diagnosis. But right now, it's my heart that is breaking and I don't really know what to do for it. Just pray, trust and depend on God. God is doing a work in me; the brokenness is leading to a new level of surrender.

Finally, on October 6, 1997—a year after our distressing trip to India and more than two years since my earliest symptoms had begun—Pamala, our good friend Dr. Lance Lee and I sat with Dr. Mastrianni to listen to the medical team's findings. Dr. Mastrianni got right to the point. He told us I was suffering from the early stages of fronto-temporal dementia.

### What is Fronto-Temporal Dementia?

**Pamala:** The term fronto-temporal dementia (FTD) covers a range of conditions, including Pick's disease, frontal lobe degeneration and dementia associated with motor neuron disease. All are caused by damage to the frontal lobe or the temporal parts of the brain or both. These areas are responsible for our behavior, our emotional responses and our language skills.

*Who is affected?* Fronto-temporal dementia is a rare form of dementia, occurring far less frequently than Alzheimer's disease, for example. Younger people, specifically those under the age of 65, are more likely to be affected. Men and women are equally likely to develop the condition.

*What are the symptoms?* Each person experiences the condition in his or her own individual way. Typically, during the initial stages, memory will still be intact, but the person's personality and behavior will change. The person may lack insight and lose the ability to empathize with others, and therefore, may appear selfish and unfeeling. A previously extroverted person may become introverted, and vice versa. The person also may become aggressive and easily distracted.

It is important to recognize that these symptoms have a physical cause and are not something the person can usually control or contain.

*What kinds of language problems occur?* The person may experience difficulties finding the right words or engaging in spontaneous conversation. They may begin exhibiting problems with circumlocution, or using too many words with too little content. Conversely, there may be a reduction in or lack of speech altogether.

*What about later stages?* The rate of progression of FTD varies enormously, ranging from less than two years to over ten years. In its later stages the damage to the brain is usually more generalized, and symptoms appear to be similar to those with Alzheimer's. Those affected may no longer recognize friends and family, and they may need nursing care.

*Is it a genetic disease?* There is a family history in about half of all cases of FTD. Some of these inherited forms have been linked to abnormalities on chromosomes 3 and 17.

*Is treatment possible?* As of yet, there is no cure for FTD, and the progression of the condition cannot be slowed.

## The Crucible and the Cocoon

**Richard:** I was buried under the load of that information for the next year. Finally, when I was able to get some perspective, I felt compelled to share some of my thoughts with my closest friends. What follows was written on the one-year anniversary of my diagnosis and sent via Email to my closest friends.

> For a few weeks now I have sensed the urge to write some thoughts about my first year in the crucible or, as I have come to see it, in the cocoon. These reflections are meant for my friends. I don't want to waste my experience. For what it's worth, I want to share them with you. My word processor and ink jet printer will spit out a neat looking document, but my experience has been anything but neat. Most of the time it has been a tangled mess. God and I are still untangling parts of my experience.
>
> On October 6, 1997, I sat in the office of Dr. James Mastrianni at the University of California in San Francisco to hear the results of hours of testing and the collective opinion and diagnosis of their research team. The news that I was suffering from the early stages of a degenerative brain disease sent shock waves through me that I still feel. Everything has changed since that day. In the words of Sue Monk Kidd, "It's anguish to come to

that place in life where you know all the words but none of the music."[1]

This is my journal entry from a few days later, Thursday, October 9:

On Monday (10/6) Pamala, Dr. Lance Lee and I were sitting at UCSF waiting for them to call my name and give their team's diagnosis. It was like the words were coming out of the doctor's mouth in slow motion. He said the words, "fronto-temporal dementia." I'm not sure if I heard "the early stages" the first time around. Dementia is a term used by doctors to describe a progressive deterioration of mental powers accompanied by changes in behavior and personality. We were given a 7-page report along with some suggestions about how to change and simplify my life. The emotional roller coaster began (as if I had not already been on one for the past year). Monday afternoon Pamala and I left for a bed-and-breakfast in Santa Cruz. We talked the rest of the day Monday and all day Tuesday. It was her love and care she showed me that somehow gave me hope as I began living my life one day at a time.

My mind has been a constant whirl of activity. I vacillate between heroic thoughts and extreme loneliness. I know I want to do what God has called me to do as long as I can, and as long as I can do it well. I want to build up my family and to make the best possible deposit in each of them with what I have left.

**Richard:** One noticeable change during this past year [1996-97] has been my reading pattern. For years I have devoured books about the church, leadership, vision and building the new community of God's kingdom on earth. All of that has ceased. Instead I find myself reading the likes of C.S. Lewis, Henri J.M. Nouwen, R.C. Sproul, Phillip Yancey and Sue Monk Kidd. You know, reflective, contemplative stuff. Stuff I didn't use to have time for. God has seen to it that I now have the time.

I have been searching for something to wrap my thoughts around or some framework on which I can connect my collection of feelings. It has come only in recent days. Out of his pastoral care for the Galatian believers, Paul revealed his heart's desire for them: "My dear children, for whom I am again in the pains of childbirth until Christ is formed in you" (Gal 4:19). The word "formed" (*morphoo*) speaks of a change of character and conduct to correspond with an inward spiritual condition. It means the internal essence rather than the outward shape. The idea is therefore of real Christlike character. Whatever else God is doing, He is forming Christ in me. Most of us, including me, prefer the sudden and painless paths to change and growth. But in creation, God has left us a number of examples of the sacred rhythm of spiritual transformation.

## The Butterfly

**Richard:** Long before a butterfly became a butterfly, it was a caterpillar. And in God's time it spun a silky cocoon or technically, a chrysalis. The transformation takes place in the chrysalis. That's where the fuzzy little creature grows its wings. Borrowing this metaphor from the writings of Sue Monk Kidd, it is this image of the chrysalis that God has pressed to my heart. This is the analogy I have searched for to make sense of my many emotions and reflections. For the past year I have been in God's chrysalis. It wasn't my idea. I went in kicking and screaming, and I'm not out yet. I have just now gotten still long enough to listen to God's voice. As I reflect on the past year, I see I have gone through a number of stages, or phases, for lack of a better term. So far I have counted seven. Let me see if I can describe them.

In the first stage, I was overwhelmed by the darkness. As a kid I was unapologetically afraid of the dark. That was before the days of Motel 6 and "We'll leave the light on." On top of that, I have always been a bit claustrophobic. As the lights went out in my world, I could almost feel the darkness. At times it was suffocating. Maybe King David was faced with his own mortality when he wrote, "You have taken my companions and loved ones from me; the *darkness* is my closest friend" (Ps 88:18, emphasis added). I don't think it has been the sheer *blackness* that bothers me most, but the inability to see beyond the immediate, the inability to chart my course. Life in the chrysalis is dark.

Even more pronounced than the darkness has been the sense of grief, the second phase of my journey. The news that I am going to die shouldn't be that alarming. Dying is a part of living. I just always thought I could die on my own terms. Stupid, huh? Right now, at least, the grief has been related to the premature end of my ministry career. I was just reaching my prime, just reaching full stride.

No doubt some of the feelings of grief have been due to my unwillingness to stay in this cocoon. For months I have felt more like I was being wrapped for burial than I was entering a cocoon. I don't feel like I have finished my course; I don't feel "done." To add grief upon grief, I feel my own farewell to my ministry has been cut short. I had my last sermons written, but I didn't get to deliver them. I didn't get to take my victory lap. For now, I have had to give up my victory lap. And to top it all off, I grieve over thinking about leaving my family.

A third stage in the chrysalis has been the sense of aloneness. I started to write *loneliness*, but I think aloneness is a better description. Pamala, my kids and my special friends have saved me from loneliness. Aloneness is the sense you feel when you are being wheeled away into surgery and everyone else must stay behind in the waiting room.

Part of the prescription that helps me function more effectively these days is a quiet environment. I have learned that aloneness is the price of that quietness. I was never one to sit still for long, so to have long periods of time by myself has been a difficult adjustment. One temptation I have had to avoid is relying on Pamala or my children to meet all my needs. The truth is, no other person can meet all of your needs. Recently I read this insightful comment: "When I lose sight of my Father/child relationship with God, I begin to look to others for more than I should. I start thinking that they are the ones who should bring me freedom, happiness and meaning. When I stop hearing God tell me that He loves me, I begin looking to others for a depth of love and affirmation that they aren't able to give."[2]

We each have to trust God and find our way through situations and circumstances that, often, no one else understands. I don't pretend to be a lepidopterist (a butterfly expert—OK, so I looked it up) but I don't think they make chrysalises for two. They are all single-seaters.

A fourth struggle has been the nagging question of "How long?" I'm neither the first—nor the last—to ask that question of God. No doubt it stems from my unwillingness to enter the chrysalis in the first place. "Haven't I already been transformed?" I ask myself. In predicting His own death and resurrection Jesus told His disciples, "Unless a kernel of wheat falls to the ground and dies, it remains only a single seed. But if it dies, it produces many seeds" (Jn 12:24). Perhaps there is a secondary application here in my situation. No doubt accepting the invitation to take up our cross and follow Jesus will mean spending some time in the chrysalis.

A fifth and predictable phase has been my struggle with the question, "What's ahead?" I don't want to misrepresent things at this point. I neither doubt nor have the assurance that God will heal me. I don't know that I will emerge from my cocoon to fly again in this life. But I do know that I *will* emerge. It may be to soar into God's presence or to continue my journey here.

A sixth struggle that recurs on a regular basis is my desire to escape the chrysalis. "What Houdini-like move can I put on my situation that will get me out of these chains?" I have always been a problem solver of sorts. Figuring things out has been my specialty. I have wanted to escape for all the reasons already cited, but I am coming to terms that there will be no escaping this cocoon. Only when God has finished His work in me will He lead me out. Sue Monk Kidd notes, "The escape hatches people create in attempts to avoid or numb pain can actually be worse than the experience of pain they sought to avoid in the first place."[3]

A way of escape was at the top of Jonah's prayer list, too. "The currents swirled about me; all your waves and breakers swept over me. I said, 'I have been banished from your sight' ... the earth beneath barred me in forever" (Jon 2:3, 6). A panic-stricken Jonah realized there was no way out unless the God who prepared the fish also prepared his escape.

The last stage to date has been the place of waiting. I have always boasted lightheartedly, "I don't *do* waiting." I have always been the kind who would eat dessert first. But God is showing me that my inability to wait is symptomatic of something amiss in my soul. Once again I share from the writing of Sue Monk Kidd: "When it comes to religion today, we tend to be long on butterflies and short on cocoons. Somehow we're going to have to relearn that the deep things of God don't come suddenly. It's as if we imagine that all of our spiritual growth potential is dehydrated contents to which we need only add some holy water to make it instantly and easily appear."[4] Ouch!

Disney World in Florida is sensitive to America's extreme resistance to waiting. A Disney employee was heard to explain that the lines to the attractions were looped and snaked to give the feeling of movement. The worst thing, he pointed out, is to let the crowd stand still. "All lines must keep moving," he said. "That's rule number one." The secret is to divert people so that they don't realize how miserable they are standing there waiting.

To me, waiting has always been a waste of time, a lack of progress, a reflection of somebody's lack of responsiveness, or the result of the "power trip" of somebody working behind a counter. I have skipped so many waiting lessons that God has decided it was time to for me to attend a crash course. George Fox called this ability to wait on God as "stayed-ness." Another has said, "When you're waiting, you're *not* doing nothing. You're doing the most important thing there is. You're allowing your soul to grow up. If you can't be still and wait, you can't become what God created you to be." God says, "Be still, and know that I am God" (Ps 46:10).

Time waiting can be time well spent. God is teaching me at least four things about waiting:

1) *Waiting is time to reflect on God's promises.* I have found it helpful to print out a list of passages from the Bible that reflect God's promise to accomplish His work in me. While I own several Bibles I can read at any time, I have found it helpful to have those promises handy.

2) *Waiting is a time to be joyful in hope.* One of the screen savers I have put on my computer displays these words of Paul: "Be joyful in hope, patient in affliction, faithful in prayer" (Rom 12:12).

3) *Waiting is a time to develop trust.* Trust may well be the believer's most important lesson. Trust is both tested and developed in the chrysalis.

4) *Waiting is a form of submission.* Submission to the Father is one of the richest qualities of a Christlike life.

### Wu Wei

**Richard:** The place of waiting is hard to describe, much less experience. Maybe it is best captured in what the Chinese call *wu wei.* It is an attitude of expectant beingness—a non-doing or actionless action that, as Thomas Merton described, "is not intent upon results and is not concerned with consciously laid plans or deliberately organized endeavors."[5] *Wu wei* is the opposite of conquest or conscious striving.

My first year of illness has left me with the understanding that my crisis is a point of separation. The word "crisis" derives from the Greek words *krisis* and *krino,* which means, "a separating." A crisis is a holy summons to cross a threshold. It involves a leaving behind and a stepping toward; a separation and a moving forward. The question I am faced with is, "What do I need to separate from and what needs to be left behind?" I only know part of the answer. That's what leads me to believe I still have some more time to spend in the chrysalis.

Crisis is also a time of opportunity. The Chinese word for "crisis" is composed of two characters. On top is the sign for *danger;* beneath is the sign for *opportunity.* This has been a time for me to "get still" so God can do His work. Getting me still hasn't been as simple as flipping a switch, but more like wrestling an alligator. But God has prevailed. I have always clung to God's promise: "He who began a good work in you [me] will carry it on to completion until the day of Christ Jesus" (Phil 1:6).

There's an old Carolina story that I like about a country boy who had a great talent for carving beautiful dogs out of wood. Every day he sat on his porch whittling, letting the shavings fall around him. One day a visitor, greatly impressed, asked him the secret of his art. "I just take a block of wood and whittle off the parts that don't look like a dog," he replied.[6]

Simple, but a good example of what God is doing in me. Pray for me, that I will embrace the full force of this opportunity to be more like Christ.

### How Do You Spell R-E-L-I-E-F?

**Pamala:** Richard was devastated by the news Dr. Mastrianni gave him that day, but my first emotion was relief. I was exhausted from the *hide-and-seek* game we had been playing for the past two years. *Hiding* the fact that Richard was ill, and *seeking* and *seeking* and *seeking* to know the cause.

However, this was just the beginning. We will share our journey in the pages that follow. We will use words to describe our journey but if you are reading this book because you or someone you love is hurting, you know mere words are not always sufficient. We have most definitely suffered physically, but the emotional toll has been far more devastating to our family. We have developed our own survivor skills, and we want very much to share these with you because we do not want our pain to be wasted. This Scripture verse means a great deal to me: "God of all healing counsel! He comes alongside of us when we go through hard times, and before you know it, he brings us alongside someone else who is going through hard times so that we can be there for that person just as God was there for us" (2 Cor 1:4, 5, THE MESSAGE).

We want to use our experience to comfort you and give you hope.

**For Group Discussion:**

1. Take 3-5 minutes and share *your* story with the group.
2. Of the seven stages of life in the cocoon (darkness, grief, aloneness, How long?, What's ahead?, desire to escape and waiting), how would you describe your current state of being?
3. Since God uses circumstances to form us, what changes can you identify as God working in you?

**Personal Application:**

1. Have you practiced the art of *wu wei* lately? What steps can you take to develop this discipline?
2. How would you answer the question, "What do I need to separate from and what needs to be left behind?"
3. Meditate on Philippians 1:6.

**Just For the Caregiver**

Few people understand the load that a caregiver shoulders daily. Can you name at least one person you can to talk with on a regular basis? If not, take time this week to list people who could possibly fill that role in your life. Then plan time with them soon. Keep it simple, but be sure to open up and share your heart with them.

# TWO

## What Will Become of Me?

**Richard:** Maybe it's a guy thing, but my identity was almost entirely tied up in what I did for a living. What I did was who I was. And I had a really good excuse to use that kind of thought process because I was in ministry. I was serving God and was valuable to the kingdom. It's that kind of nonsense that fuels the notion that God loves me because of what I do for Him. But I am disappointed to confess it has taken me a full three years since I learned of my illness to come to grips with this issue.

### My Story

One fall afternoon after my diagnosis I was sitting in the office of a Christian psychologist and he asked me that famed question, "Tell me, how are you feeling these days?" I had grown accustomed to the routine of his questions, so I had thought ahead of how I would answer on this particular day. I told him I saw myself, along with all my family and friends, standing around on a large iceberg. But as I watched, the ice upon which I was standing broke away and I began to drift away from those I loved, isolated on an island. I'm not sure where the image of the ice came from, but the sense of separation was a cold reality. Things were not the same; they could never be the same.

After my diagnosis, in an attempt to stay in my role as senior pastor of the church where I served, I arranged for other staff members to take over some of my responsibilities. This seemed to work for a few months, but the plan quickly deteriorated. Things were changing and they were out of my control. That was something I wasn't accustomed to. I could no longer lead, I could no longer cast vision, I could no longer problem-solve, and I could no longer do the very things I felt God had gifted me to do.

At first, I had a sense I would die within a year's time. After all, without my identity, what was the use of hanging around? Or was there another option? Perhaps God would fashion in me a new identity, albeit temporary.

After I resigned my position at the church, Pamala and I had to give consideration to relocating to a more economical location. California on a full wage was tough enough, but California on a disability payment was simply impossible. Pamala and our daughter, Amy, surveyed the options and we decided to move to Oklahoma. Since Pamala was born in Oklahoma and her parents lived there (as well as one of my sisters), it seemed like a logical move.

So in July 1998 we moved to the Tulsa area. Notice I said *July*. It took much of the month. While a mover hauled our belongings the fifteen hundred miles, our family flew one way to Tulsa. When this California boy stepped off the plane and into the summer heat and humidity of Tulsa, immediately I wondered what I had gotten myself into. I wanted to go back—*back* to my old life. I didn't want things to change. I loved my life. But there was no going back.

Don't get me wrong. I have grown to like Oklahoma, but there is not a day that goes by that I don't miss my life, my former identity. Here nobody recognizes me. Here nobody knows of my accomplishments in life. Here nobody knows who I really am. I am left with my diplomas and certificates to hang on my bedroom wall for no one to view except myself.

At first I felt compelled to make people aware of who I was, or at least who I had been. But somehow that felt inappropriate. I concluded I would just have to establish a new identity—a new scaled-down model. With the help of family and friends I came to realize that while I grieved over the past, I was wasting present opportunities. Indeed, there is a time and place for grief but it can easily become a permanent stranglehold rather than the temporary phase it is meant to be.

I have learned there are different kinds of grief. Being in ministry for thirty years I have performed numerous funerals and have tried to console those who lost loved ones. When a loved one had lived a long and full life, even though people grieved, they would often say, "We knew it was coming." There was time to prepare. There was almost a sense of expectation and, on some occasions, even relief.

But in the case of a long, lingering illness, the grief seems to be endless—like being in slow motion. At what point should we give up hope? At what point should we grieve? Should we mask our grief? Those are questions my family and I must grapple with on a daily basis. For me, I felt like I was drowning. I did not want to die even though I knew things would never be the same. And being the stubborn person I am, if I couldn't have it my own way, then nothing else would do. But that left me in a quandary, with an option I was unwilling to accept. My suffering has made me much more aware of others around me who suffer as well.

**A New, Smaller World**

While driving my car one fall afternoon in 1998 I heard a radio commercial advertising a Christian college that offered a degree program for working adults. It piqued my interest—maybe I could teach there, I thought. I did a little searching on the Internet and located the website for Bartlesville Wesleyan College (now Oklahoma Wesleyan University). I found the Email address for the academic dean and submitted online a resume and a brief description of my circumstances. To my surprise I received a phone call from the director of the program. He wanted me to come to his office for an interview.

That was the beginning of a year-long relationship with an outstanding Christian college and community of staff and students. The classes were one night a week, and I was able to keep pace with that kind of schedule. For a period of several months, Pamala or someone else would drive me to the school, then pick me up and take me home.

Eventually, I had to resign my position due to the fact that I no longer have the endurance to teach a four-hour class. It was taking me up to two full days to recover. Once again, I felt a piece of me slipping away. Again, I was losing control.

In January 2000 the church we attended began a new venture. In addition to the two Sunday morning services it already had, the church decided to begin offering a Saturday night service. They asked if I would do the preaching. I took on the project with my usual enthusiasm. But I had to take precautions I was not accustomed to. Previously, I had had an experience on a Sunday morning when, about five minutes into my message, I could not speak—I just froze up. I looked down at my notes and saw the words, but somehow my brain would not send the necessary signal for my mouth to move. I had to excuse myself, and Pamala helped me off the stage and took me home.

In this new endeavor I worked hard to prevent that from happening again. I scripted out my messages word for word. Pamala would sit on the front row with a copy of the manuscript and coach me if I came to a place were I would lose my train of thought. I served in that capacity for one year, but eventually had to give that up too.

Again, I have had to face reality. I could no longer, for lack of a better term, "make things happen." And frankly, that has been a good thing. I had been accustomed to "making things happen" in ministry. That's the way to get the "atta boys" and slaps on the back. The truth is, my identity needed purging.

God is not impressed (nor was He ever impressed) with my ability to make things happen. Part of what God is teaching me is that I matter to Him no matter what stage in life I find myself. So how can I hold myself to a higher standard than God does? I will cease to be what I once was, but at the same time I can become what God intends for me.

People who participate in Make Today Count groups (an organization for people with terminal illnesses) often speak of a syndrome they label, "pre-mortem dying."[1] In effect it is an advanced case of helplessness. Gradually, inexorably, everything that has given a person a sense of place, a role in life, is taken away. Dr. Eric Cassell, an internist at Cornell University, concluded about his patients, "If I had to pick the aspect of illness that is most destructive to the sick, I would choose the loss of control."[2]

One of the horrible things about illness—terminal illness—is that it robs us of our identity. When I was a pastor people knew me everywhere I went. Not only that, but my wife and children also drew their sense of identity from the fact that I knew who I was and they belonged to me. As my world was unraveling, so was theirs.

## Loss and Discovery

**Pamala:** Loss will affect everyone's life in some way. Our loss as a family was clear: we lost Richard in the role we knew him in. I met Richard when I was fourteen at church camp. We grew up together. I was in awe of him from the very start. He was tall, good-looking, very intelligent, strong and a determined Christian leader. We dated for five years and then got married. I scarcely have a memory that does not include Richard.

Because I married so young, I must admit, I did not completely develop my own separate identity. I was Richard's wife and the mother of three. I believe I excelled in those roles. I was happy to look after Richard, believe in him, cheer him on and support his dreams in life. I loved to watch him each Sunday behind the pulpit as he spoke with wisdom and authority. I learned so much of the Bible from his proficient teaching. He was in a class of his own, blessed and gifted with communication expertise. My part was to make certain he looked good, and felt very much loved and satisfied. He did and was, so I felt fulfilled. This, plus being a mom, was my highest calling in life. I took pride in both. I focused on Richard and the kids, knowing and loving their uniqueness.

If I would choose metaphors to describe each of our lives,

it would look something like this: Richard's life would be a *race*. He was always in a hurry and he definitely wanted to win. My life would be a *dance*. Music is imperative in my life. Sometimes fast, sometimes slow, it is always passionate and emotional—just like me. Apryl, our older daughter, is a *party*. She loves a crowd, noise, motion and commotion. Amy, our younger daughter, is a *classroom*. She lives to learn more, achieve more and get an A+ at whatever she does. Aaron's life would be a *stage*. He loves being on the center of it, and he loves to entertain and make everyone laugh.

As I assess our group of five, I see how God designed our family perfectly for what we are going through presently. In our crisis, we have all needed something besides dad's "race" to keep us going. Apryl has a husband and four children; her life is a constant "party" of six. Amy is back in the college "classroom" seeking her second degree, this time to become a chiropractor. Aaron is on "stage" in a Christian punk band, writing, rehearsing and performing. I am a deejay on a local radio station while, at the same time, writing this book. I wake up each morning to music, "dance" to it throughout the day and fall asleep listening to it every night. Music keeps me company during long hours of being alone. God has provided perfectly for all of us during the unanticipated journey we are now on.

Discovering and staying true to our own identities has been a process. Richard's illness set that into motion. The illness, though tragic, has in a positive way challenged me to reach goals I would never have even dared to set before. I am back in college after thirty years and am a 4.0 student. I have invested in stock, made money, purchased and sold real estate on my own, painted murals in our home, as well as at several businesses in town. I have met many new friends who have never met Richard and they actually like me for just me—I wasn't sure that was possible. One more thing: I now choose my favorite types of dancing where, before, I would always follow Richard's choice, which was always fast, perfect and proper.

I know God wants us to find whatever good we can from what we see as the bad in our lives. I feel our family is doing pretty well at this. I have lost a lot, but I have discovered that what I miss the most is the history I have with Richard: the memories, the one-liners, the inside jokes that no one will get but him. The fact that he was there when our babies took their first breaths, attended their first days of school, hit their first home runs, became first-time drivers, and when we had our first grandchild.... I know no one will ever share these same memories with me. But it is comforting to know that what I miss is something I can always hold in my heart, that nothing can take away, not even when Richard is gone from us.

## A Positive View

**Apryl:** I am the oldest child, so among us three kids, I have the most memories. Now I am a grown woman with children of my own, but I still remember when my sister, Amy, and my brother, Aaron, were born. Being the oldest, I was the first to try everything! That was good and not-so-good at times.

My dad and I have had a typical dad-and-daughter relationship throughout the years. You know, I drove him crazy, but he was crazy about me anyway. That's what I have chosen to focus on throughout this journey we've been on with Dad. I look back positively at what I have had, not at what I have lost.

These are the positive things I think about:

- I had a dad growing up. I choose to be thankful for that time we shared.
- My dad's last act of fathering me was the most significant in my life. I needed him to help me get into a drug and alcohol rehabilitation facility. He found the best one and made certain I got into it. It was only a few months later that he was forced to resign from his church and move to Oklahoma.
- I must depend on God as my Father now. The Bible says that God will be a Father to the fatherless. I claim that promise often. I trust God's infinite wisdom at this stage of my life and of my dad's.
- I choose to accept my mom's decisions in Dad's care since I do not live near them. I have said good-bye to Dad many times, and each time, I hope to see him again in this life. Each time, I know it may not be here but in heaven that I see him again. I know he will be happy and not suffer there, so I give these uncertainties to God and His will.

My biggest regret is for my four children. I wish they had their Poppy Richard around. The older girls do have good memories with him, but my baby boys really do not even know him. But I still see how I can turn this into a positive. I can learn to savor my time with my children, hoping they are storing up memories with me that nothing can ever take from them, like my memories of my dad. None of us knows for certain if we have another day, month or year with our loved ones.

One thing my parents taught me and lived before me was that God is our Father and He is always there. I turn to Him for everything these days. If I have a question I might have asked my dad, I now ask God. God is a great listener and an excellent parent. He actually doesn't let me get by with some things my dad would have, but then I am sure there are things even God lets slide because He loves me so much!

## All in This Together

**Amy:** Growing up, I remember people asking me what it was like to have a dad like mine—a teacher, pastor and respected leader. The question always puzzled me because he was my father and had been all those things as far back as my memory reached. I would respond by saying, "Just normal, I guess."

As I got older, however, I began to realize it wasn't exactly normal. Not only would we get recognized when we went out as a family, but people knew who I was even when Dad wasn't around. His position and status in the community was apparent, and somehow I felt I was an extension of that.

When Dad was first diagnosed, I was in my early twenties. As we began to learn and understand what the prognosis of the disease would entail, it was obvious that my dad was going to have to resign his position as senior pastor. I can only guess how difficult that must have been for him personally. But it wasn't so much the change of his position in the community that affected me as much as it was the change of his position in our family.

It was difficult for my dad to talk to us about his disease even though my sister and I were both grown. It also became more difficult to seek out my dad's advice regarding other areas in my life. We could only imagine the personal state of turmoil he must have been living through and so we tiptoed around him. I did not ask him for fatherly direction or guidance so that I would not add to his burden.

But in addition to my Dad's diagnosis, it was also a difficult time for me personally. Not only was I was in the "trying-to-define-myself" stage of life, but I also became involved in a difficult relationship. Instead of adding to my parents' stresses by asking for help, I let myself think I could handle it on my own. I tried to be more adult than I was ready for and I made some wrong choices. I learned several things the hard way, but most of all, I learned that a family will be there for each other regardless of other circumstances.

My biggest struggle with Dad's illness has been that we didn't talk about it openly and candidly in the early stages. I am sure this would have been very difficult for all of us, but I believe it would have kept the family communication open— not just about the disease, but about other issues affecting our lives as well. My mom was the one that kept me informed. But I wanted to be more of a part of things, and I think talking about it earlier would have been therapeutic for all of us.

We talk about things now. I think it just took us a while to realize it wasn't just Dad being affected by this disease, but we all had to deal with it. It may affect us differently— Dad with the actual symptoms, Mom as the primary caregiver, and the rest of us as supporters—but we did realize we were all in this together and became a closer family because of it.

It can still be difficult when I think about the fact that my dad may not watch me graduate as a Doctor of Chiropractic, and that he probably will not see my children born, watch them grow up and have their own accomplishments. I some-times even become so selfish that I ask God to let him stay with us. But, I know in my heart that we are all a part of God's plan. I might not always understand it, but that's not my job; my job it to trust God and know that underneath all the sadness and tears there is hope because I will see my dad again, together with my heavenly Father.

## Never Give up Hope

**Aaron:** I'm nineteen now. When my mom told me my dad was sick I was fourteen. We were eating at a McDonald's in our town in California and she started being weird, talking about how high school was going to be different in Oklahoma. But I didn't see how, other than the move and the differences in the states, so I kept questioning her. I wanted her to elaborate on what she was talking about. After that, she said that dad was going to die, perhaps even before I graduated.

My first reaction was that she was obviously crazy because graduation wasn't very far away. She explained that they had caught Dad's illness a few years into the disease, and we were pressured to relocate due to a reduction in his income.

After moving to Tulsa I wanted to push away all the reality my family was trying to feed me. No one wants to dwell on the fact that his dad is dying when there isn't a single thing he can do about it. I always wanted to think things were getting better and Dad was doing well. I guess I was just deluding myself.

Things did seem to get better; my dad was sitting right next to my mom and my girlfriend on the night I graduated from high school. The ceremony took a lot out of him so he didn't go out to dinner with us afterwards.

I knew that my dad easily grew tired and was distracted by noise and commotion. It didn't help when I had friends over to the house, and we were loud and noisy. After my senior year my dad moved away from the noise to a place of his own at a retirement center. It has been good for him, but he admits frequently that he is lonely there.

I have caught myself ditching him for my stupid friends. "Hello, idiot! Spend time with your dad!" It wasn't that I didn't want to be around him; even his being sick didn't bother me one bit. He likes to hang out with me; I make him laugh and everything is OK for a while.

I love my father more than ever right now, and not just because he's sick and I won't get to hang out with him in the future. My parents have taught me to NEVER GIVE UP HOPE IN CHRIST! I recently read through the book of Jeremiah and it restored so much hope in me. "Heal me, O Lord, and I will be healed; save me and I will be saved" (Jer 17:14). "'But I will restore you to health and heal all your wounds,' declares the Lord" (Jer 30:17). I am trusting Christ for my future and the future of my father.

However, sometimes God allows bad things to happen to His children. This is where "God's plan" comes into play. Everything happens for a reason. My dad got sick and it affected our family a lot. But it has caused positive things to happen: 1) I have found my relationship with Christ has grown in trusting Him for all my needs; 2) My sisters' lives have become more focused and they too see what God has planned for them through all of this; and 3) Mom and Dad have had the opportunity to write this book so other people can find hope and encouragement in Christ. There can be so many reasons this "bad thing" is happening to my dad. So I can say to you without any doubt: DO NOT GIVE UP HOPE IN CHRIST! He will never let you down. In my times of hardship and trials He has made His plan apparent and how I am to follow His Word.

My God is a jealous one and wants ALL of me. Not just some or certain parts or in certain situations—He wants ALL of me. I have surrendered my life to Christ. I have given up worrying and questioning "why?" Once you learn to cast every care you have on God (1 Pt 5:6-7) your heart will be new with no worries, no cares. You will be able to trust His will—that in the end all will work out according to His plan and purpose. I have submitted to the fact that His ways are higher than ours. He will bring about good through our family's trials and that is OK with me.

**For Group Discussion:**

1. Do you sense that your world is "shrinking"? Can you share an experience with the group?
2. Discuss Dr. Eric Cassell's comment, "If I had to pick the aspect of illness that is most destructive to the sick, I would choose the loss of control."
3. What do you think Jesus meant when He cried out to His Father, "My God, My God, why have you forsaken me?"

**Personal Application:**

1. Read and reflect on Psalm 73. What was David experiencing at that time in his life?
2. Do you have a trusted friend or group of friends? If not, ask God to bring someone into your life to walk with you.
3. How is God reshaping your identity? Does it need purging in any way?

**Just For the Caregiver**

There is a constant threat of getting so caught up in the daily care of the person you are caring for that you neglect to live life. Make a point today to do something that has nothing to do with being a caregiver. (And do not feel guilty!) Often caregivers feel guilty about taking some time for themselves. Maybe this week you can go to a movie, a concert or something you enjoy. Treat yourself well, spoil yourself momentarily and keep your emotional tank full.

# THREE

## What Is Suffering?

**Richard:** Pain and suffering are all around us. According to one report, one in three people in America live with chronic pain or chronic illness. I actually thought in the back of my mind I could run the gauntlet and not be touched. How could I have been so naive? I may be a saint in the New Testament sense of the word, but I have found that I am no superhero.

Before my illness, the pain I was most accustomed to was the physical kind. My introduction to physical pain as a youth was when I would fall off my High Flyer and skin my knee, or I would hit a rock while riding and go sailing through the air. I would come down on the asphalt pavement skidding on my back—*without* a shirt! That was my introduction to pain—and to iodine. For the most part I have learned how to avoid pain that is physical in nature. However, for many, physical pain comes knocking at your door without an invitation. Some of you have to plan your life around your physical pain and my heart goes out to you.

But pain comes in other forms as well. Emotional pain is another major source of suffering in our world. I, for one, have become more familiar with emotional pain than I would have ever dreamed. Who's to say which type of suffering is more painful? It's not a contest to be won or lost. On a daily basis I give thanks to God that my suffering does not—as of yet—involve physical pain.

## Pain Is an Intruder

**Richard:** Pain—whatever kind it is—by its very definition inflicts discomfort. Much like a pebble in our shoe that causes us to limp, pain causes us to change our behavior, and sometimes our future. Pain is never fair. It takes aim at the young and the old alike. And it can be a dream robber. It can take the best part of us and leave us to wonder, "What might have been?"

Though my disease has been "painless" in the physical sense, it has brought a laundry list of things that hurt. I think what I hurt about most is that I don't feel *finished*. I was never much of an athlete, but I've heard professional athletes who have their careers cut short often report this same kind of disappointment. I felt I was at the top of my "game," and then—without warning—the game was over. I am grateful I can still write an hour or two a day, write letters to those in prison and pray for people around the world, but the one thing God called me to do—and equipped me to do—is over. I still feel a God-sized passion in my heart, but it is housed in the body of a helpless child.

## Pain and Suffering Keep Us From Moving

In his book *A Grace Disguised,* Gerald L. Sittser, who lost his wife, his mother and a daughter in a head-on collision, writes of his struggle to make sense of tragedy:

> Loss creates a barren present, as if one were sailing on a vast sea of nothingness. Those who suffer loss live suspended between a past for which they long and a future for which they hope. They want to return to the harbor of the familiar past and recover what was lost.... Or they want to sail on and discover a meaningful future that

promises to bring them life again.... Instead, they find themselves living in a barren present that is empty of meaning.[1]

**Pain and Suffering Cause us to Compensate**

I am left-handed. Part of my brain disorder has caused my left side to have tremors—especially in my hand. As a result I have had to learn how to write with my right hand. It has felt like being in kindergarten all over again. It has been embarrassing to write a check at the grocery store in the check-out line. I could hear the sighs of people as they waited in frustration for the "old guy" to write his check. Now I have actually gotten pretty good with my right hand and have learned to fill out most of the check before getting in line! But that is a small compensation compared to what others—maybe you—have endured. Pain forces us to find another way.

**A Side Effect of Suffering is Depression**

Depression has been called "the common cold of mental health problems." Consider these facts:

- More than 5 percent of Americans—some 15 million people—suffer clinical depression at any given moment.
- Another 5 percent experience mild symptoms of being "down in the dumps."
- At least one person in six experiences a serious, or "major," depressive episode at some point in life.
- Each year, tens of thousands of depressed people attempt suicide. About sixteen thousand succeed. Suicide is now a leading cause of death among teens and young adults.[2]

I remember when I was told that I was suffering from depression. I rose up out of my chair in objection and assured the doctor that I was very optimistic about the future and was not bummed out about anything. Then he explained the difference between clinical depression and situational depression. I learned a lesson that day. Clinical depression is triggered in the sufferer by a chemical imbalance or physiological cause. Situational depression, on the other hand, is triggered by a circumstance or something that happens to cause a person to feel helpless, hopeless and depressed. This is what I was suffering from.

## Pain Exposes Need

**Richard:** I am a slow learner, but I am being "schooled" on the fact that pain and suffering have an upside as well. To be honest, I almost choke on those words. But think about it, pain is what often sparks much of our music, art or literature. After meeting Pamala during a week at summer camp at the age of sixteen, my heart was so distressed by our separation that I wrote her a twenty-three-page letter. That was the beginning of my writing career! The pain of separation caused me to pour out my heart to her.

Without pain, our world might have little of the scientific knowledge or technology we have today because many of inventions and discoveries are made as a result of a need. To be without pain is virtually to be without need.

## Pain Evokes the Fight/Flight Response

While some of us want to run at the first sight of pain or trouble, I believe most people want to fight for self-preservation. It is not in our instinct to give up without a fight. But to fight requires courage. So we look for a source of courage. I recently read, "Courage is fear that has said its prayers." That's worth taking note of, if I do say so myself.

Pain and suffering are also closely related to what the Bible calls perseverance or endurance. Endurance is steady determination to keep going even when everything in you wants to slow down or give up. The apostle Paul went so far as to say, "We also *rejoice* in our sufferings, because we know that suffering produces perseverance" (Rom 5:3, emphasis added). How could he say such a thing? The idea of suffering here has the underlying meaning of being under pressure; it was used to describe squeezing olives in the press in order to extract the oil or of squeezing grapes to extract the juice. The pressure brought to bear has a purpose in mind: in the case of olives, producing oil; in the case of grapes, juice. In your case and mine, God is seeking to "squeeze" the characteristics of endurance, hope and love.

### Endurance

**Pamala:** This journey of suffering has changed me forever. Now I have true strength of heart, soul and body. Before I had always just tried to appear to be a superhero, complete with a big red "S" on my chest. No one knew that under my superhero suit resided a scared wimp. In true hero form I would press ahead regardless of the crisis, never revealing my true identity. I was compelled to appear superhuman—it was my trademark. I was, after all, the daughter of a minister, a 4.0 student, wife of a successful pastor and a mother. I was determined to exude absolute perfection, meeting everyone's expectations with my superhuman powers like all faith-filled people do.

Surprisingly I got through many incredible challenges. It looked as if I was pulling it off, but in reality I was weakening with each new crisis. Still, I refused to remove the big red "S" from my chest. I felt if I appeared weak it would be a bad reflection on my faith and on God's strength. I had a lot to learn about appearances—that just appearing strong is a poor stand-in for true endurance.

Endurance is what it takes to get through a long haul. To endure means "to suffer patiently without yielding; to last; to continue in existence." Endurance is not developed quickly or effortlessly. Any facade of super humanness has to go. You cannot fake it. If you try faking it, you just won't last.

Our long haul would be a degenerative brain disease, a slow but steady death for Richard and a journey of suffering in slow motion for our entire family. We all needed endurance.

Endurance is an inside job and that was my problem: "inside" was hard for me to find. I had spent my time perfecting the big red "S" on the outside for all to see. No one, including me, was looking inside. However this new crisis hurt so much, was so deep and frightening, and so hopeless, I was forced to rip the big red "S" from my chest. This left a hole in my humanity, but it also created an entrance to the innermost part of me.

Finding the inside of me is what saved me. I didn't realize that the big red "S" was really a prison from which I needed to be set free. Although I would never have chosen suffering to gain my freedom, the truth is, I now am free. It did not happen overnight and there were days I wanted to wimp out. I even wished for my fairy godmother to come with her magic wand and change me instantly, but no wand appeared. Instead I rested and sought God for new courage. I found I was going to have to work at this soul-finding thing. God, not a fairy godmother, would be there to strengthen my steps, *but it was my job to take the steps.* I have listed five steps here and trust they can help you as you develop the endurance you will need for your long haul.

1. *Seek solitude.* As long as there is distraction you will not have the discipline it takes to look deep within. I went away for a week by myself. I rented a cabin in the Santa Cruz Mountains. I took food, my Bible and a journal. No phone, no television, no computer, no work, and the most difficult for me ... no people. I am a people addict. Yes, there is such a thing. I despise being alone. But I needed to be alone so I would be forced to talk to myself.

2. *Talk to yourself.* Ask questions you would ask someone you want to know intimately.

- How would you describe yourself?
- What is the best thing about you?
- What is your greatest failure?
- What do you want said about you when you are gone? Will it be said?
- Who do you trust? Why?
- Who are your heroes? Why?
- What do you really want to do with your life? Are you doing it now?

- What would you change if you could?
- Make a list of the top five priorities in your life. Do you give them priority?
- What is the worst thing that has ever happened to you?
- What do you consider your greatest accomplishment?
- What brings you the greatest joy?
- Do the people you love know it? Are you sure? How can you be sure?

I wrote the answers to these questions in my journal. I soon realized I wanted far more out of my life than I was getting. I needed to make a lot of changes.

3. *Make a list of the things you need to change.* When someone wants to get stronger physically they must stop doing certain things, like eating junk food, and they start doing other things, like eating healthy and exercising. The same process has to happen with emotional fitness. There are things to stop doing and things to start doing.

4. *Make a list of things you want to start doing.* I decided to go back to college. I needed to know how to be on my own. There was a lot to learn and I was behind. I also wanted to start having some fun in my life. I wanted to do things that were *my* idea of fun, not my kids' or Richard's idea of fun, but mine. I also wanted to broaden my base of friends.

Friendships are a necessity for the long haul of suffering. I discovered I needed about five very loyal, trustworthy friends to aid me on the journey. I had only two when we began six years ago. I now have numerous acquaintances that care *a little* and five friends who care *a lot.* I say without hesitation the care they have given me is definitely divine. I prayed for God to send me kindred spirits who would love me through this and He did. You will need friends. I advise asking God to send them to you. He chooses perfectly.

5. *Get to know God intimately.* I knew *about* God all of my life. But through our suffering I got to know God. Knowing about Him is not enough in the dark hours of the night. There will be times when there is no one, not even the closest of friends, who can relieve the deep pain you are experiencing, who can give you hope when there is none in sight, who can bring peace and comfort to your aching heart. God and He alone has the power to do all of this and more. He has made me sing and dance in the darkest of nights. He has never left me alone on this journey and I know He will not let you down if you take the time to get to know God intimately.

You will need endurance for your journey ahead. I am thankful for the strength I now possess inside—strength of heart, soul and body.

### Pain and Suffering Bear Witness to a Genuine Faith

**Richard:** But God cannot bring about this desired quality of endurance without our cooperation. "Consider it a sheer gift, friends, when tests and challenges come at you from all sides. You know that under pressure, your faith-life is forced into the open and shows its true colors. So don't try to get out of anything prematurely. Let it do its work so you become mature and well-developed, not deficient in any way" (Jas 1:3,4, THE MESSAGE). Do you see the emphasis there—*let* pressure do its work. Building a persevering spirit is not a passive matter. It takes courageous participation on our part as we work in cooperation with God.

Paul tells of a time when he was under great pressure, so much so that he feared for his life. But in retrospect he could later write, "But this happened that we might not rely on ourselves but on God" (2 Cor 1:9). It matters to God that we find our sufficiency in Him.

"In this you greatly rejoice, though now for a little while you may have had to suffer grief in all kinds of trials. These have come so that your faith—of greater worth than gold, which perishes even though refined by fire—may be *proved genuine* and may result in praise, glory and honor when Jesus Christ is revealed" (1 Pt 1:6, 7, emphasis added). You might ask, "Doesn't God already know if our faith is genuine?" Yes, of course He does. But you and I need to know what we're made of. We need to be assured that our faith is solid and grounded in a genuine relationship with God.

Oliver Cromwell was Lord Protector of the Commonwealth of England, Scotland and Ireland during the dark days of civil war in the mid-seventeenth century. During Cromwell's administration, the treasury ran out of silver that was used to mint coinage for the realm. Cromwell sent some of his men to travel throughout the kingdom and find silver for the treasury to use.

The delegation reported back to Cromwell that the only silver they could find was in the statues of the saints in the cathedrals. "What should we do?" they asked their leader.

Cromwell replied, "We will melt the saints and put them into circulation."[3]

In much the same manner, before God can use a person,

before He can put His servants into circulation, He has to put them through a meltdown. If you are facing a meltdown, rest assured that God is not attempting to destroy you. Much like the smelting process, God's refining fire purifies us and is His instrument to test our "metal," to purify us and to bring glory to Himself by making us better people.

I can testify to the fact that suffering can bring about a purifying process in our lives. Of course, I'm not saying that all suffering is brought on by our sin, but it causes us to look inward and invites us to accept the challenge to "come near to God" (Jas 4:8).

To say that suffering has an upside is not to minimize the *real* nature of pain and suffering. I don't know if I'm ready to jump up and down and say that suffering is worth the exchange for character development, but I do know I am a better person and I like myself more now than the person I was before.

**For Group Discussion:**
1. Is your suffering mostly physical, emotional, or both?
2. Can you share with the group one of the dreams that pain and suffering has robbed you of?
3. Pamala offers five steps to developing endurance. Which step do you need to focus on most at this present time?

**For Personal Application:**
1. How has your suffering purified your life?
2. Pamala suggests that you "talk to yourself." Work through the questions she poses and record your answers in your journal.

3. Endurance requires we cooperate with God. Are you resisting Him in any area of your life? If so, why?

## Just For the Caregiver

In this chapter Pamala talks about the value of solitude. Granted, solitude is not everybody's favorite pastime, but on occasion solitude can be a source of refueling. Every day we need a few minutes of solitude, whether it is to pray, meditate, read the Bible or just enjoy the quiet. Weekly we need to break away for an hour or two just for time to be alone. But once or twice a year, like Pamala described, we need to take as much as a day or two to go away and leave our televisions and telephones at home (OK, maybe take a cell phone to check in once a day). Look at your calendar and make plans to get away. Use that time to review the thirteen questions she outlines and to journal your responses.

# FOUR

## Trading Fear for Trust

**Richard:** Jesus and His disciples were bone tired. He suggested, "Come with me by yourselves to a quiet place and get some rest" (Mk 6:31). Jesus made His disciples get into the boat and go on ahead of Him. But when they were in the middle of the sea the winds rose up against them. Many of them were former fishermen so this was no big deal, right? Wrong.

Jesus could see them from the mountaintop where He was praying: they were "straining at the oars" (v. 48). That expression arrests my attention. I suppose they could have rowed all night and made safe passage to the other side, but Jesus came to them—walking on the water at about the fourth watch (3:00-6:00 A.M.). "But when they saw him walking on the lake, they thought he was a ghost. They cried out, because they all saw him and were terrified" (6:50). They did not recognize Him and were more frightened by His presence than by His absence.

### Don't Be Afraid

Jesus said, "Take courage! It is I. Don't be afraid" (6:51). Mark's explanation is that Jesus "wanted to pass by them" (6:48, literal translation). Some have suggested that Jesus was sneaking up on them to playfully surprise them. I don't think so. Others have explained that Jesus was simply rescuing His frightened disciples. Either way, when Jesus planned to pass by His disciples—who were straining at the oars—He wanted them to see His majesty as the Son of God and to give them reassurance. His mere presence caused the wind to cease howling and enabled the disciples to continue their journey.

Like the disciples, I know how it feels to be afraid of my circumstances and to do the first thing that comes to my mind—row! Just as a drowning person thrashes about in the water, a person who is filled with fear "strains at the oars." Are your hands calloused from too much time on the oars?

No matter what you are suffering, fear is probably and will continue to be a factor. I read the following story in *Our Daily Bread:*[1]

> One night during a thunderstorm, a mother was tucking her young son into bed. She was about to turn the light off when he asked in a trembling voice, "Mommy, will you stay with me all night?" The mother gave him a warm reassuring hug and said tenderly, "I can't, Dear. I have to sleep in Daddy's room." After a brief pause, the boy replied, "The big sissy!"

### That Four-Letter Word: F-E-A-R

**Pamala:** Fear. It's such a small word, yet it carries a power so intense it can grip and paralyze each of its victims. The anxiety it produces can become a monster lurking just beneath the surface of our lives. In his book, Archibald Hart notes, "Anxiety's one creative facet is that it feeds on itself. Legitimate concerns can turn into worry. Worry becomes anxiety and anxiety can dominate life."[2] Anxiety causes us just to sit, stew and become stressed out, all the while robbing us of joy and peace. When we are prisoners of fear we become completely miserable, unable to live life with any joy or hope.

During fearful times we may have thoughts like, "You are all alone," or "God can't handle this problem," or "God could care less about your crisis." These thoughts cause us to doubt God's love and involvement in our lives. But God is able. We can have faith that He is big enough to handle any problem— including *our* problem. Our mistake is to focus on the hopeless circumstances instead of on God's power to help!

Scripture reminds us: "See, the Sovereign Lord comes with power, and his arm rules for him.... He tends his flock like a shepherd: He gathers the lambs in his arms and *carries them close to his heart;* he gently leads" (Is 40:10-11, emphasis added). I know this is a reality. I have felt Him carry our family close to His heart.

The only power over fear is complete trust and rest in God. Have you noticed it is impossible to trust and worry at the same time? The usual pattern is to volley back and forth between the two at first, and then give in to one of them.

**Trust For the Storms of Life**
When I was a little girl in Oklahoma we had tornado season every spring. It was on one of those cool, quiet May evenings that I learned an important lesson in trust.

Our family was sitting at home this particular night. We lived in the parsonage right next door to our church. Daddy was reading, and my big brother, Larry, was working on a model airplane while I was coloring a glorious picture of springtime flowers. Mom was busy getting my baby sister,

Debbie, ready for bed, when suddenly, without any warning, the wind and rain started pounding against the big picture window in our living room. Within moments my mom and daddy were tuning into the local radio station for a weather report. With concerned brow, my mom began to gather up blankets, coats and my baby sister. Soon our phone began to ring with calls from concerned neighbors, urging my dad to open the church basement for shelter. The basement was the neighborhood storm cellar. Everyone—sinner and saint— would gather underneath the giant brick church building when a storm came up.

This was a *real* storm—not just a warning! The weatherman said a tornado had been sighted and it was heading straight for our little town of Wewoka. Everyone was urged to seek shelter—and fast!

My dad grabbed the keys and headed to the church with my brother right behind him. Others met them in our yard; all were hurrying to the basement. My mom held my baby sister tightly as she threw a blanket snugly over her. She headed out the door of our home. As the wind grabbed at her on the porch, I heard my instructions. "Wait here until Daddy comes back for you; the wind is too strong."

There I stood, alone, in the middle of the deserted house, eagerly waiting for the sight of my daddy to take me to safety. Soon, the tall familiar figure I knew and trusted stood in the doorway. My dad had come to take me to safety. He took me by the hand and said gently, "Pam, do not let go of my hand, OK?" He didn't have to worry. I wasn't about to let go. I'm sure the perspiration on my sweaty little hands had instantly turned to superglue.

As we stepped outside into the darkest of night, I could feel the hard rain beating down upon me. The wind was fierce, tearing at my coat. Then we heard it! It was the deafening sound of a tornado. I could see its gray funnel winding up toward the sky as it headed straight toward us!

"Hold on Pam. Hold on baby. Daddy knows the way. Just don't let go of my hand." Within moments we were safe inside the old basement. My dad motioned toward an old table. "Pam, go sit under that old wood table. I want you to stay there until this storm passes over."

It was cold and uncomfortable, not to mention boring, under that old wood table. But I knew the storm was tearing things apart just above us, and that my daddy had brought me to a safe place. I had trusted him as we ran through the pouring rain to get here, and even though it was most uncomfortable, I stayed under that table for a long, long time that night. I wasn't really worried; I trusted my dad's wisdom and knowledge of tornadoes. I chose to rest and not be afraid.

Since then I have endured many storms in my life. Some have been emotional, some spiritual, others physical, but all of them have been scary. Through each of them I have learned that if I hold tightly to my faith in God and trust Him to guide me to safety, I can find rest, even comfort, during the roughest of storms.

During fearful anxious times it takes the letting go of fear and the taking hold of someone's hand to lead you into the safe and restful place. Sometimes it's the hand of a trusted family member or friend. Other times it's taking hold of the unshakable hand of God to lead you into peace of heart and mind.

## Five Common Fears

1. *Fear of going to a place you have never been before.*
**Richard:** I remember the day they slid me into an MRI tube. MRI is short for magnetic resonance imaging. The procedure is an imaging technique used primarily in medical settings to produce high quality images of the inside of the human body. My doctors were looking for the possibility of a brain tumor in the early stages of my diagnosis. It was one of the most unpleasant experiences I have ever had. You've heard the saying "one size fits all"? Well that isn't true when it comes to an MRI tube. This tube seems made for a small woman and I am an extra-extra-large man! Lying inside of it, my body was touching the sides of the tube everywhere. They told me to be still; I couldn't have moved if I wanted to.

They also told me the machine would make some noise as it took the images of my brain. This must have been the old model because it sounded like it could throw a rod at any moment. Right above my eyes was a small mirror that allowed me to see my toes and the nurse that stood behind the plate glass window during the procedure. Oh, did I tell you I am claustrophobic? This was not a pleasant experience. We had to break up the lengthy procedure into several shorter segments that day so I could come out of the tube for short breaks. (Now I know what it feels like to be a burrito.)

My point is that we all tend to fear "parts unknown" and going places that are unfamiliar. When we feel a sense of panic come over us, we tend to "strain at the oars."

2. *Fear of not knowing what the future holds.* It took more than a year for the doctors to give me a diagnosis, and then they

weren't absolutely positive. Somehow I felt that if I knew what was wrong with me, I could attack it as I had any other project. But test after test and doctor after doctor could not come up with a conclusive diagnosis. The guys in the white lab coats are supposed to know everything, aren't they? Not knowing for sure was killing me.

My mind worked overtime to come to some sense of understanding of what was happening to me. During this time I had a dream—or maybe it was a vision—that I believe gave me a sense of insight into what was happening to my health.

Every home has an electrical panel. It's usually located in the garage or in some remote corner of the house. Mine is located in my laundry room directly between my washer and dryer. The panel is usually rectangular in shape and gray in color. When you open the door there is a main switch and two columns of circuit breakers.

In my dream the door of the panel opened and I looked inside. I saw that the main breaker was in the "On" position. But one by one the circuit breakers were being switched to the "Off" position. When I woke up I realized that was what is happening to me. The electrical current is the source of life. To switch the main breaker to the "Off" position would bring death. But the same result can be achieved by turning off the circuit breakers one at a time.

The human brain is a lot like the electrical panel in your home. Although the brain is much more complicated, the image of the circuitry applies to my illness. I am grateful to still be alive, but there is no doubt that my circuit breakers are slowly being switched to the "Off" position. Let me see if I can illustrate it. If a circuit breaker that controls the electrical current in your kitchen were turned off, the outlets in your bathroom would still work. You might even conclude that nothing is wrong with the electrical circuits in your home—until you attempt to use your microwave oven.

Let me make this more personal. I have often had people tell me that I seem "fine" to them. There are times I can carry on normal conversation and spend time writing a book. What they don't know is that when I am in a restaurant and there are conversations going on all around, my brain cannot filter out the background noise and allow me to focus on the person I am talking to. They don't know that I have lost 75 percent of my "horsepower" and energy to perform tasks that were once simple. They don't know that I sometimes lose my balance and have suffered a partial loss of vision in one of my eyes. They don't know that my left hand shakes too much to write a check so I have had to learn to write with my right hand. And these are small issues compared to many others who suffer from this disease. For me my symptoms will get worse in time. For others, they are already at advanced stages.

3. *Fear of death.* Fear is a natural emotion. It's part of the fight/flight response. But if left unchecked fear can paralyze us. Facing the reality of our mortality can be among the most fearful things we will ever experience in life. Part of the process of courage is identifying our fears. That's exactly what I decided to do one afternoon. I turned on my computer and decided to list "My Fears." For what it's worth, I want to open up my heart and let you see what I feared on that particular day.

- It makes me afraid to know that Pamala will marry another man. Of course she will be free to do so, but for some reason I fear the fact that I will not be able to share that part of her life. I met Pamala when I was sixteen and married her when I was twenty. I just can't imagine life without her.

- I will miss significant events in the lives of my children and grandchildren. Of course this is the concern of every parent. We naturally want to enjoy all of the birthdays, graduations, weddings, births and baptisms of every one of our children and grandchildren. For me, it's easy to focus on what I will miss rather than dwell on all of the wonderful experiences I treasure.

- I fear that my death will be long and drawn out. I fear the whole idea of suffering in slow motion.

- I dread the boredom often associated with this kind of illness. I am sick enough to be disabled but well enough to feel miserable when I am unable to be active.

- I fear I will become a burden on my family. Pamala and I have agreed in prayer that if God does not choose to bring healing that He will take me home to be with Him rather than suffer a long, drawn-out death.

- I fear the isolation that illness brings. I already sense it and I know it will only increase with time.

There are those who would tell me I shouldn't be afraid, and maybe they're right. But what I *should* feel and what I *do* feel are not always aligned in a way I would like.

The next part of my exercise in identifying my fear was to search for God's antidote. I like the way Rich Mullins expressed it in his song, *Hold Me Jesus:*

Sometimes my life just don't make sense at all.
When the mountains look so big,
And my faith just seems so small.
**Chorus:**
So hold me Jesus 'cause I'm shaking like a leaf.
You have been King of my glory,
Won't you be my Prince of peace.

(Rich Mullins ©1993 Class Reunion Music)

God knew that we would often suffer from fear. Lloyd Ogilvie notes there are three hundred and sixty-six "fear not" verses in the Bible—one for every day of the year, including one for leap year! Most of the "fear not" verses have to do with God's presence with us in the midst of our fear and trouble. For example, consider this promise:

When you pass through the waters, I will be with you;
And when you pass through the rivers, they will not sweep over you.
When you walk through the fire, you will not be burned;
the flames will not set you ablaze.
For I am the Lord, your God,
the Holy One of Israel, your Savior.

ISAIAH 43:2-3

After making my own personal list of fears I took it to God. Then I turned my *fear* list into my *prayer* list. For every fear God reminded me of His goodness and provisions in my life. He reminded me of the memorable years of marriage with Pamala. He reminded me of all the memories of three wonderful children and four grandchildren. I even laughed out loud as God reminded me of some of our family vacations! It's easy to always want more.

In the place of fear I am asking God to give me the attitude of gratitude. Honestly, I struggle with it some days. Some days I revert to the mode of wanting what doesn't seem to be God's plan for me. But then along comes a reminder of gratitude. Gratitude can deal a deadly blow to fear.

### 4. *Fear of failing.*

**Pamala:** For family and friends of the terminally ill person there is a constant nagging in the soul reminding them that the one they love is dying. Of course we all will die at some point, but it is very different when you have been told the process has begun in someone you love. I try not to dwell on this fact too much, but it does disrupt my thoughts on a regular basis. I know there will be a day when Richard will be gone from our lives. One of my ongoing fears is having enough energy to last, enough patience and love to keep giving. I want to finish well—you know, no regrets in this long good-bye.

Admittedly there are advantages in having time to say good-bye to your loved one, but there comes a point when you become exhausted from the very long and drawn-out good-bye. You just want all the suffering, all of the daily grieving, all of the letting go to be final. This may seem selfish to someone who did not have an opportunity to say good-bye to a person they loved in the way they wanted to. But to those who have watched the daily, inch-by-inch death of the one they love, it seems more merciful. I fear wearing out, of becoming weary in well-doing, or not finishing this challenge courageously. I fear that when I look back, I will wish I had done it better, or given more.

But living in fear is a waste of time. Fear robs all of us of needed rest. It robs us of peace. We need to cherish the time we have and not worry over the "what ifs." This will rob us of living life today.

My way of combating my fear was somewhat different than Richard's. I had to admit it existed and talk to someone about it. When I finally had enough courage to tell my friend Cheryl about this fear she was completely shocked at my jaded perception. She brought to light the many times I had found strength when I thought I had none left. She reminded me of the patience and love I had shown Richard in very difficult times. Cheryl and others could see the tenderness and care our family was giving to Richard when we had lost sight of it.

I realize now that many of our fears prove to be invalid. Most things we fear never come about. I encourage you not to waste energy on fear. Allow yourself to be human. You will disappoint yourself from time to time, but when you do, remind yourself of these things:

- All the care you are providing now.
- All the love you have given.
- The tenderness you have shown all along the long journey.
- The days and nights of praying for your loved one.

Don't worry about small defeats along the way. Every person dealing with a lengthy illness will grow tired, frustrated and feel overwhelmed. I have learned to live one day at a time with Richard's illness. I cannot take on the end when it is not here. While he is here I will try to do the best I can and not fear those things that have not even happened, and I doubt ever will.

Our family has said good-bye to Richard a hundred times. As he is left with less and less of his life, we grieve over his loss—and our loss. Watching this giant of a man become weak and frail, awkward, fearful, disconnected, confused and needy is not easy. This has turned into a long and very sad good-bye to someone we love and miss every day.

Richard has expressed his desire to leave this life with some dignity left and we want this for him as well. But this is out of our control; it is in the hands of God. Accepting this takes a heart that trusts in God's love for each of us. God has placed us in a position of dependency on Him and we are learning to trust Him. It has not been an easy lesson. From the onset of Richard's illness our family realized that this suffering in slow motion was going to take supernatural strength—God-sized strength. And it is taking a lot of trust.

5. *Fear of fault or blame.*
**Richard:** Underlying the question "Why?" is the question "Whose fault is this?" It is so easy to get trapped in the revolving door of "if only." If only I had taken better care of myself; if only I had paid closer attention; if only I had prayed harder, believed more; if only, if only. Somehow we think if we could attach blame then we would feel better about our circum-

stances. But rarely can blame be affixed. Maybe it can in the case of a drunk driver or a homicide, but so often the cause of our suffering has no culprit.

This brings me back to the picture of Jesus and His disciples on the water that night. All our fears can lead us to row harder. At least when we are rowing we are doing "something," right? But maybe we should entertain the thought that Jesus wants to "pass by us." Perhaps He wants to reveal Himself to us in a way we have never known Him before.

## What Is Trust?

**Pamala:** Getting back to the topic of trusting God, trust is the opposite of fear. I believe trust is a process: the more someone proves to be trustworthy, the more trust is possible. It takes a great deal of trust to lean into a Person I cannot physically feel, pray to ears I do not see and trust hands that I cannot touch to provide. But I can say without a moment of hesitation that God has proven absolutely trustworthy each time I have trusted Him with my needs.

What does it really mean to trust? It cannot be defined easily and it is even harder to put into practice. Webster defines trust as, "Assured reliance on the character, ability, strength, or truth of someone or something"; "having confidence placed in one"; or "something committed into the care of another." OK, that's the definition of the word as a noun. But you and I both know that trust is also a verb: It requires action. Trust is a deliberate act we choose to do or not to do. Through my own process of learning to trust, I developed an acrostic to help me better define the true nature of trust:

**T**aking hold of God's hand and *letting go of what's in mine.*
**R**esting *instead of wrestling.*
**U**nconditional love for God, *even when I don't understand Him.*
**S**urrender my will to His. *Dying to self is very hard to do.*
**T**iming; accepting God's timetable as perfect, *regardless of how long.*

When there is pain and suffering in our lives, we have a choice as to how we will respond. We can choose to get angry, depressed and hurt by the pain and allow ourselves to become a hard and hollow cynic. But I believe that even through the painful, despairing times of life, it is possible to become a more loving and compassionate person. The key is to choose to trust God with our pain.

There is much peace in trusting God's love and care with our lives and the lives of our family. Webster's says trust is an assured *reliance* on the character, ability, strength, or truth of *someone....* There is no greater *Someone* to rely upon than the Creator of the universe. I cannot see Him, but I have felt His presence. It is like the wind I cannot see, yet I know it is there because of what I see it do and how it makes me feel.

I have felt God's presence close to me and I have seen Him do some incredible things. For instance, God has provided for us financially throughout Richard's illness in a very creative way. We had been on staff at several churches during our thirty years of ministry, but only one provided sufficient disability insurance to care for Richard if he should become disabled: it was the last church where Richard pastored. This particular insurance pays us for as long as Richard lives—with no reduction of benefits. Because of this, for six years now I have been able to take care of him and the family without having to seek outside employment. We did have to relocate to a less expensive area to live, but even in the experience of relocation we have seen God's plan for our family unfold.

Time after time, there have been answers to specific prayers we have prayed—things only God could accomplish. But the most undeniable evidence of His love and presence is the instant peace He has given us—at times, for no other reason except we asked Him for it. I know it was from Him because the pain we felt was so great no person could have eased it, and no amount of money or pleasure could have provided that kind of comfort.

Only by calling out to God has peace come to us in our pain. Just like the time Jesus calmed a raging storm and brought perfect peace simply by His command (Mk 4:39), so He has done with us. God has personally calmed my rage, my pain, my loneliness and my fears by trusting in His power to do so. Try it. It works! You will see that He is absolutely trustworthy in everything. But you must first be willing to trust Him.

**For Group Discussion:**
1. Can you identify what causes you the most fear? Can you share it with the group?
2. Can you remember your earliest childhood prayer?
3. Which part of the T.R.U.S.T. acrostic speaks to your most present need? Can you share it with the group?

**For Personal Application:**
1. Does God want to *pass by* you? What is He saying?
2. List your fears and search for corresponding promises in God's Word. Keep this handy for future reference.
3. Journal your thoughts about your fears and any growing sense of trust you have in God's promises.

**Just For the Caregiver**

Today is the day to remove the big red "S" from your chest and admit to being human. List your honest fears, talk them over with a close friend and in prayer give each one of them to God. If trusting God in this way is new for you perhaps today is the perfect time to experience the peace He gives when we ask Him for help.

## Part II

## I WILL FEAR NO EVIL

# FIVE

## Keys to Living with Loss

**Richard:** Sooner or later all of us will experience loss. The question is, "How will we live with our loss?" We have no control over how much we lose or how often we lose, but we do have control over how we respond. I would like to offer a few practical ways of approaching life that will help us remain positive even in the face of loss.

1. *Live with expectancy, not expectation.* I was sitting in church listening to the pastor give a message titled, "What to Do When Life Seems Diminished," when he said something that has stayed in my mind ever since. He made a distinction between living with expectancy and living with expectation. "Expectation tends to dictate terms to God,"[1] he explained. He went on to say that expectation insists that God do things my way and in my time frame. Expectations are our attempts to put God on our time schedule and to work according to our demands. To live with expectation is to set ourselves up for disappointment because even the most casual Bible reader knows that God is sovereign and doesn't operate this way.

Expectancy, on the other hand, is the belief that God will do something: It is always looking out for what He will do. Living with expectancy allows God room to work, but in His way and in His time. This way we cling to the promises of God without holding Him hostage to our demands.

2. *Get some much-needed perspective.* I suffer from tunnel vision. Not literally, but in a very real sense. I tend to see only my immediate circumstances and what is right before my eyes. I often lack the broader view of what's going on in my life. It's a matter of perspective, the lens through which we choose to look at the things that matter most.

Fortunately for people like me, perspective is available from a number of sources. For me, the Bible is my foremost source. The psalmist writes, "Your word is a lamp to my feet and a light for my path" (Ps 119:105). I can go there to find out the truth about whatever I am facing.

Friends can be a source of perspective also. They can be a "sounding board" for us. "As iron sharpens iron, so one man sharpens another" (Prv 27:17).

Solitude has also long been a practice of people trying to gain perspective through the centuries.

Another of my favorite sources of perspective is reading. While reading is sometimes taxing to my mind, it can also be refreshing and delightful. It provides another lens through which we can look at the world. Take for example this story I read recently:

> The story is told of a man who loses his wife. He is devastated and seeks comfort. He travels to an old woman in the village who, he has heard, holds the answers to life's great questions. He tells her of his loss and his pain. The woman sits quietly, listening to the travail of the bereaved husband. Then she responds, "There is a plant that can cure the pain of loss. But it must be specially grown. In order to grow it, you must find a mustard seed from a home that has known no loss."

The man sets out eagerly on his quest. He soon discovers that each home he approaches has a tale of woe. He returns to the woman and says, Now I understand. There is no home without loss. The woman smiles gently.[2]

3. *Hold on to your hope.* Usually hope is focused on the future. The Bible says, "But hope that is seen is no hope at all. Who hopes for what he already has? But if we hope for what we do not yet have, we wait for it patiently" (Rom 8:24-25). While grief may cause us to look back, hope tugs at our hearts to look to the future. Let me give you an example.

Viktor Frankl was a Viennese psychiatrist who survived the Nazi death camps at Auschwitz and Treblinka. His work and experiences are documented in his book, *Man's Search for Meaning.* In it he concludes that the primary force in our lives is, in fact, our search for meaning, and hope plays a key role in this. While in the concentration camps, he discovered that the prisoner who no longer had a goal in life was unlikely to survive:

We who lived in concentration camps can remember men who walked through the huts comforting others, giving away their last piece of bread. They may have been few in number, but they offer sufficient proof that everything can be taken away from a man but one thing: the last of the human freedoms—to choose one's attitude in any given set of circumstances, to choose one's way. The way in which a man accepts his fate and all the suffering it entails, the way in which he takes up his cross, gives him ample opportunity—even in the most difficult circumstances—to add deeper meaning to his life."[3]

Frankl further describes how living without a sense of hope posed the greatest difficulty for the prisoners:

> Former prisoners, when writing or relating their experiences, agree that the most depressing influence of all was that a prisoner could not know how long his term of imprisonment would be. He had been given no date for his release. A well-known research psychologist has pointed out that life in a concentration camp could be called a "provisional existence." We can add to this by defining it as a "provisional existence of unknown limit."[4]

Frankl tells of two would-be suicide cases that were averted. While many prisoners ended their own lives despite the efforts of others to talk them out of it, at least two prisoners were successfully reasoned with because they had something to live for. "We found, in fact, that for the one it was his child whom he adored and who was waiting for him in a foreign country. For the other it was a thing, not a person. This man was a scientist and had written a series of books, which still needed to be finished. His work could not be done by anyone else."[5]

While I don't subscribe to all of Frankl's theories, he makes many good points. Hope is essential to our ability to go on. For those of us in the midst of suffering and loss, having expectancy, perspective and hope can all be lifesavers. These three keys will help you survive when you feel your world has crashed in around you. They can help you change your focus from your present set of circumstances to what is around the next corner.

## What a Way to Go

**Richard, as told to Pamala:** Recently, just before the church service began, I overheard two people behind me talking about a family member who had recently died in his sleep. "What a way to go," one said. The other person replied, "When it's my time, that's the way I want to go."

Some people die peacefully in their sleep; others are tragically killed in accidents. And then there are those who battle and struggle for years with a disease that kills them one day at a time.

I think we Americans have this notion that if we eat our veggies and lay off the junk food we deserve to live until we are a hundred. But I have known a lot of "healthy" people who have died. The Bible cautions us repeatedly about assuming we have all the time in the world.

*Teach us to number our days aright, that we may gain a heart of wisdom.*

PSALM 90:12

*Now listen, you who say, "Today or tomorrow we will go to this or that city, spend a year there, carry on business and make money." Why, you do not even know what will happen tomorrow. What is your life? You are a mist that appears for a little while and then vanishes. Instead, you ought to say, "If it is the Lord's will, we will live and do this or that."*

JAMES 4:13-15

While it may be an unpleasant thought, we are all in line—in line to die. Our thinking is that the old should die first. If the young die, we often refer to it as a "premature" death. Somehow we think we all deserve a long and healthy life. Any aberration from our plan is an assault on our sense of justice and fairness. God owes us that much, doesn't He? But while we are all in line, some of us get our "number" called and we move to the head of the line.

### Exit Plans

Assuming we could choose the way we exit this planet (and that is a huge assumption), how would you want to go? If I haven't already lost you, I hope you will stay with me a little longer. Here are some alternatives from which to choose.

### Plan A

First is what I will call Plan A. This is one we don't see that often. According to all known medical research, the current death rate is 100 percent—minus two, that is. The Bible tells of two men who did not die a natural death. You may already know their names: Enoch and Elijah. But let's take a closer look. Chapter five of Genesis is not exactly a thriller; it is a list of the genealogy from Adam to Noah. You know: so-and-so begat so-and-so, etc. And then we come to this statement: "Enoch walked with God; then he was no more, because God took him away." In the case of every other person mentioned in Genesis chapter five, his life ended with, "and he died." Everyone but Enoch. Enoch's walk with God was not a fifty-yard dash; instead he walked with God for three hundred years, and then God took him away. The word used in this case means, "to carry away, to fetch, or to send for." What a way to go!

Elijah was the Old Testament prophet of fire. This guy ate nails for breakfast. He spoke the truth before kings (not to mention that he ran from their wives). He challenged the false prophets of Baal to a litmus test involving fire from heaven, saying, "The god who answers by fire—he is God." Talk about sticking your neck out. But Elijah also had a propensity for depression. When he wasn't calling down fire from heaven or swatting the Jordan with his mantle, he seemed more human than the superhero we make him to be.

However, Elijah accomplished his mission. (What joy there must be in knowing that you have served your God-given task in life, that you have fulfilled your destiny!) One afternoon as Elijah and his protégé Elisha were walking along, God sent His chariot of fire and horses of fire to escort Elijah into heaven, "and Elisha saw him no more."

Plan A is pretty cool, huh? What a way to go!

## Plan B

Plan B is an event on a much larger scale than Plan A. While Plan A was personal and individual, Plan B is personal but massive. While the odds of Plan A happening might be very small, the chances of you and I being a part of Plan B is much higher. But maybe I'm getting ahead of myself.

Plan B is that event in the future when "the Lord himself will come down from heaven, with a loud command, with the voice of the archangel and with the trumpet call of God, and the dead in Christ will rise first. After that, we who are still alive and are left will be caught up together with them in the clouds to meet the Lord in the air. And so we will be with the Lord forever" (2 Thes 4:16-17). Millions of people, all around the world, will be caught up to meet the Lord in the air. Millions of people will not face natural death! The word used to describe this event means, "to catch up, to pluck, to pull, or to take away." The Latin word used is *rapture*. A discussion on the timing of this event is beyond the scope of this chapter, but the point is, Plan B is still in the future and millions of people will go directly to heaven without having to die! What a way to go!

I confess I prefer either Plan A or Plan B, but I have to be honest with myself and realize the choice is not mine to make. None of us knows what tomorrow holds, so we may have to consider yet another plan.

## Plan C

Plan C is again personal and individual. It is modeled for us in the life of another person of antiquity—a man named Jacob. As his life drew toward its end, Jacob gathered his children around him so that he could bless them and tell them what would happen to them in the days to come. One by one, he spoke words of blessing and words of caution to his children. What a tragedy when mothers and fathers die leaving unfinished business with their children. This lack of closure haunts many people I know. I am determined to bless my children often so that whether I go via Plan A, B or C (or via some other plan), they will have a recent memory of a blessing I spoke to them.

Jacob also gave his family instructions about his burial. Though they had lived for many years in Egypt, Jacob wanted to be buried in Canaan, the land of his fathers. What enormous pressure we put upon our spouses or children when we fail to communicate our desires about burial. What a simple exercise it would be to write out your desires for your burial and memorial service, and put it away in a safe place.

I thought to myself, "If Jacob were alive today, how would he communicate his wishes and blessings to his family?" My guess is that he would take the time to contact an attorney and draw up a Living Trust. He would bless his family with treasures and mementos of his affection for each of them. He might make a videotape to be played as the family gathered after his death. He might even set up a website where he would post lots of pictures of his grandkids. The Bible tells us, "When Jacob had finished giving instructions to his sons, he drew his feet up into the bed, breathed his last and was gathered to his people" (49:33). What a way to go!

If my guess is right, we all intend to do some of the above-mentioned ideas, but we just never seem to get around to it. The important is rarely urgent. But more valuable than an inheritance is the gift of a blessing. That's the way to go.

I know my time is drawing near. I am still hoping for Plan B, but I know that Plan C is a very real option. Maybe I should plan for C, but hope for B. I think that's what I will do. I know the Lord could return at any moment, but if not, I must be prepared to deal with the realities of living and dying.

### Jacob's Model

Recently I drew up a document that I titled "My Wishes." Using Jacob's case as a model, I tried to think through a series of questions and came up with plans concerning my memorial service. Pamala and I have already had a Living Trust drawn up, but this involved even more specific details concerning the last chapter of my life on this earth. Some of the questions I considered were:

1. To whom do I give the responsibility of carrying out my wishes? I don't want to put added pressure on Pamala so I have asked one of my dearest friends to coordinate my memorial service and events related to it.

2. What about the actual funeral and burial arrangements? Pamala and I have already met with a local mortuary to make our decisions now so that there will be no pressure or anxiety when the time to die comes.

3. Who do I want to thank? This is a big deal to me. Many people have contributed to my life. The list could have gone on and on, but I have assimilated a list of people who influenced me the most. I want that document read at my memorial service.

4. What about the memorial service itself? I have decided that my family and closest friends will be invited to a graveside service that will precede the memorial service. I want the memorial service to be a celebration—a celebration of the life God allowed me to live, and a celebration of the gift of eternal life through Jesus Christ my Lord. I have even selected music and burned it onto a CD that will be played in the memorial service. Planning the service is my way of "attending" the service. What a way to go!

**For Group Discussion:**

1. Why do you think so many Americans have become health conscious?
2. Which is better: to live a *long* life or to live a *godly* life?
3. What are some ways we can *bless* our children and grand-children?

**Personal Application:**

1. Do you feel that God *owes* you smooth sailing in life?
2. Using Jacob's model, how should you prepare for your future?

**Just For the Caregiver**

Even though it is not easy to think of "Final Wishes," remember "terminal" does mean that one day someone will be faced with making hard decisions for your loved one. If your loved one can share in these decisions as Richard did, then set up a time to talk about them in an open and honest way. Perhaps you could use Richard's list as a guideline to help pave the way into this very difficult subject. If he or she is not able to take part in this discussion, then perhaps another family member could assist you as you make these plans in advance. Do not wait until the end, when everyone is distraught and emotions are frail.

## SIX

## When God *Doesn't*

**Richard:** I like it when God steps in and saves the day, don't you? It makes me cheer when I read about God's angels showing up in the lion's den to rescue Daniel. In fact, God's list of rescues in the Bible is pretty impressive. One could be led to assume God *always* saves the day. But does He? What about the times when God *doesn't?*

### When God Does Not Rescue

We are all familiar with scenarios in life when God did not rescue people from tragedy. What about the mother and father who ask God to heal their child from a terminal disease, and He *doesn't?* What about the children who kneel beside their beds at night and ask God to give Daddy a new job or to stop him from hurting Mommy, but He *doesn't?* What about the wife who asks God to protect her police officer husband, and he is killed in the line of duty? What about the missionaries who have given their lives to spreading the gospel and are killed by the very people they are trying to reach with the life-giving message of Christ?

What about stories like this one I read:

**Killer Wind Shakes Town**

PIEDMONT, Ala.—This is a place where grandmothers hold babies on their laps under the stars and whisper in their ears that the lights in the sky are holes in the floor of heaven.

This is a place where the song "Jesus Loves Me" has rocked generations to sleep, and heaven is not a concept, but a destination.

Yet in this place where many things, even storms, are viewed as God's will, people strong in their faith died last week in, of all places, a church.

"We are trained from birth not to question God," said twenty-three-year-old Robyn Tucker King of Piedmont, where twenty people, including six children, were killed when a tornado tore through the Goshen United Methodist Church on Palm Sunday.

"But why?" she said. "Why a church? Why those little children? Why? Why? Why?"

The destruction of this little country church and the deaths, including the pastor's vivacious four-year-old daughter, has shaken the faith of many people here. It is not that it has turned them against God. But it has hurt them in a place usually safe from the hurt, like a bruise on the soul.

They saw friends and family crushed in what they believed to be the safest place on earth, then carried away on stretchers of splintered church pews.

But more troubling than anything said the people who lost friends and family in the Goshen church, were those tiny patent-leather children's shoes scattered in the ruin. They were new Easter shoes, bought for church.

"If that don't shake your faith," said Michael Spears, "nothing will." Others are confused. "It was church," said Jerri Kernes. "It isn't supposed to happen in church."[1]

That expression, "a bruise on the soul" has stayed with me. What do we do when life turns out differently than we plan? Or when things don't turn out as we hoped? Or when we continue to suffer? What do we do when God *doesn't?* I once read, "God needs no defense—but people often need an explanation."

I can assure you I don't have all the answers. In fact, I have more than my share of unanswered questions. But I'd like to offer some new perspective I've gleaned from reading numerous books on the subject of suffering.

### If Only We Knew "Why?"

There have been many treatises, both ancient and modern, that have tackled the subject of why people suffer. Somehow, we reason, if we could master this subject, we might be able to step closer to accepting why we, or people we love, are not spared from suffering. We keep searching for the "why" because we really want some control over our lives. But God doesn't always grant it.

"There comes a time in every life when all hell breaks loose,"[2] writes Steven Lawson, in his book by a similar title. He explains:

There is something about our inquisitive minds that long for answers. If only we knew why, we reason, then we could handle the pain. But let's face it, even if God were to explain to us all the whys, we couldn't understand it. Placing His infinite wisdom into our finite brains would be like trying to pour the Atlantic Ocean into a Dixie Cup.[3]

But however true this may be, it doesn't keep us from wanting to know why, does it?

One survey reports that, of 139 tribal groups from around the world, all but four of them perceive illness as a sign of God's (or god's) disapproval.[4]

But the confusion doesn't stop there. The faith of many people has been shredded by the "why" question. Perhaps your own faith has been stretched to the limit by your trials.

Author James Dobson has said, "My concern is that many believers apparently feel God owes them smooth sailing or at least a full explanation (and perhaps an apology) for the hardships they encounter."[5]

One thing is for certain: our faith will not go unchallenged for long. And there is no guarantee we will ever understand why.

Consider the case of Rabbi Harold Kushner.

### Is God All-Powerful?

I have reread Rabbi Harold Kushner's book *When Bad Things Happen to Good People* for the third time. It is acclaimed as a bestseller that has brought peace to millions. Kushner is no stranger to suffering. His son, Aaron, at the age of three was diagnosed with a condition called *progeria*, or "rapid aging." The doctors told the family that Aaron would never grow much beyond three feet in height, would look like a little old man while he was still a child, and would die in his early teens. Aaron died two days after his fourteenth birthday.

Kushner says that he and his wife had grown up with the image of God as an all-wise, all-powerful parent figure who treated us as our earthly parents did, or even better. If we were obedient and deserving, He would reward us. If we got out of line, He would discipline us, reluctantly but firmly.

Kushner poses many questions in his book, then provides a number of options for why good people suffer. First, he explores the view that we deserve what we get in this life. Next he asks if suffering can be educational. Can it cure us of our faults and make us better people? He frowns upon the literal translations of verses such as Proverbs 3:12, "For whom the Lord loves, he chastises, even as a father does to the son he loves." Thirdly, he looks into the notion that all tragedy is some form of cosmic test. "If God is testing us, He must know by now that many of us fail the test. If He is only giving us burdens we can bear, I have seen Him miscalculate far too often."[6]

After posing these questions, Kushner launches into the ancient story of Job. "Job was so good, so perfect, that you realize at once that you are not reading about a real-life person. This is a "once-upon-a-time" story about a good man who suffered." Kushner asks, "What kind of God would that story have us believe in, who would kill innocent children and visit unbearable anguish on His most devout follower in order to prove a point, in order, we almost feel, to win a bet with Satan?"[7]

Kushner goes on to propose three statements:

A. God is all-powerful and causes everything that happens in the world. Nothing happens without His willing it.

B. God is just and fair, and stands for people getting what they deserve, so that the good prosper and the wicked are punished.

C. Job is a good person.

The rabbi asserts that as long as Job is healthy and wealthy, we can all embrace these three statements. But when Job suffers, when he loses his possessions, his family and his health, we have a problem. If God is both just and powerful, then Job must be a sinner who deserves what is happening to him. If Job is good but God causes his suffering anyway, then God is not just. If Job deserved better and God did not send his suffering, then God is not all-powerful. And so his logic goes.

Kushner's book is a sad read. In his search for solace he has decided that the words of the Bible cannot be taken literally: "No matter what stories we were taught about Daniel or Jonah in Sunday school, God does not reach down and interrupt the workings of laws of nature to protect the righteous from harm."[8] While it is not my purpose to take the gloves off and go after Kushner, I wonder what kind of peace one can experience believing in a God who is not all-powerful or one who doesn't intervene in our behalf?

Author Phillip Yancey weighs in on this matter and suggests that there are two great errors that commonly corrode our thinking. The first is the error of attributing all suffering to God. The second error does just the opposite, assuming that life with God will never include suffering.[9] Either extreme will lead to disillusion and disappointment.

Going back to Job, his case is second to none among human loss and suffering. But, for what it's worth, there is something in it that is often overlooked. Though Job lost everything—his children, his wealth, his servants, his reputation and his friends—this was not the source of Job's most intense frustration. Listen to Job's anguish: "If only I knew where to find him; if only I could go to his dwelling! I would state my case before him and fill my mouth with arguments. But if I go to the east, he is not there; if I go to the west, I do not find him. When he is at work in the north, I do not see him; when he turns to the south, I catch no glimpse of him" (Jb 23:3-4, 8-9). One of Job's greatest frustrations, it seems, was his inability to find an audience with God. Much of his suffering was from not being able to reach God in his distress.

## A Christian Perspective

No Christian treatment of suffering would be complete without looking into what Jesus said on the subject. Jesus' disciples asked, "Who is responsible for suffering?" The clearest insight into that question appears in Luke, chapter thirteen. Jesus declares that Satan caused the pain of a woman bound in disease for eighteen years.

Early in the same chapter Jesus is asked about two other events that were taking place at that time. One was an act of political oppression in which Roman soldiers slaughtered members of a religious sect; the other was a construction accident that killed eighteen people. Jesus never explains why, but He makes one thing clear: they did not occur as a result of specific wrongdoing. "Do you think that these Galileans were worse sinners than all the other Galileans because they suffered this way? I tell you, no!... Or those eighteen who died when the tower of Siloam fell on them—do you think they were more guilty than all the others living in Jerusalem? I tell you, no!" (Lk 13:2-5). (He doesn't say so, but maybe this tower was built by the lowest bidder.)

Jesus doesn't stop His lesson there. He implies that we "bystanders" of catastrophe have as much to learn from the event as do the victims. A tragedy should alert us to make ourselves ready in case we are the next victim of a falling tower or an act of political terrorism.

In these passages, we see the disciples looking backward to find out "Why?" much like we do today. But Jesus redirected their attention. He pointed forward, to the concept of preparing themselves. In doing this He answered a different question: not the "Why" but "To what end?"

However we look at suffering, we will all experience it at one time or another. The question is not so much "Why?" as it is "What will we learn from it?" and "How will we deal with it?" Will we break and run? Will we throw in the towel? Will we "curse God and die," as Job's wife suggested to him? Ultimately, the question is "How?" or "To what end?" rather than "Why?"

### The Product of Suffering

While I am in no hurry to run to the head of the line, suffering produces something. It has value; it changes us. The biblical command for us to take joy or to rejoice in our suffering is not suggesting that Christians should act happy about tragedy and pain when they feel like crying. Rather, the Bible aims the spotlight on the end result, the productive use that God can make of suffering in our lives. Pain and suffering are part and parcel of living in a fallen world. While there is much we do not know about suffering, we can focus on what we do know.

God has many reasons for allowing us to suffer:

- Suffering silences Satan (Jb 1–2).
- Suffering gives God an opportunity to be glorified (Jn 11:4).
- Suffering can make us more like Christ (Phil 3:10; Heb 2:10).
- Suffering can make us more appreciative (Rom 8:28).
- Suffering teaches us to depend on God (Ex 14:13-14; Is 40:28-31).
- Suffering enables us to exercise our faith (Jb 23:10; Rom 8:24-25).
- Suffering teaches us patience (Rom 5:3; Jas 1:2-4).
- Suffering can make us sympathetic (2 Cor 1:3-6).
- Suffering can make and keep us humble (2 Cor 12:7-10).
- Suffering brings rewards (2 Tm 2:12; 1 Pt 4:12-13).

I was diagnosed with my illness at the age of forty-eight. My first thoughts were no doubt the same as many of yours. Why *me?* Why *now?* My birth certificate did not come with a guarantee that I would live to be eighty. My hope is in the promise of eternal life for all who have placed their trust in Jesus Christ. My prayer is that God will help you see above your present trials, trust Him with your unanswered questions and be able to focus on His promises.

## Coming to Terms With When God *Doesn't*

No matter how much we search for answers, in the end, we must interpret the unknown in light of the known. Allow me to share some of my thoughts about when God *doesn't*. I believe there are four things we can be sure of:

1. *It is never because He cannot.* Our God is able (Mt 3:9, Jude 1:24, Eph 3:20). You name it and God can do it. One agnostic argued that, given the presence of evil in the world, God is either not omnipotent or not loving (or good). If evil exists because God does not want it to exist but is unable to prevent it, then He is not omnipotent. If He is omnipotent but allows it to exist, then He is neither loving nor good. Either way the presence of evil is fatal to Christianity, according to the agnostic.

When God fails to live up to our expectations it is not because He is not strong enough to bring it to pass.

2. *It is never because God doesn't love us.* God's love for His children is unconditional and enduring (Jn 3:16; Rom 8:35, 37-39). God has demonstrated His love and our worth to Him by giving His only begotten Son to reconcile us to Himself. God's activity—or inactivity—is never motivated by anything but His love for us.

3. *It is never because we are unworthy.* God has never done anything for us on the basis of our worthiness or denied us anything on the basis of our unworthiness (Rom 10:4). The basis for His activity in our lives is always His grace—period!

4. *It is never because He is not committed to our best welfare.* God has the same disposition toward us as He had toward Israel and His promise is still good: "I know the plans I have for you," declares the Lord, "plans to prosper you and not to harm you, plans to give you hope and a future" (Jer 29:11).

So how are we to understand the times when God doesn't heal, doesn't fix, doesn't intervene, and doesn't take away the pain?

First of all, when God *doesn't*, we should view His response in the light of what we know about His character. Understanding the character of their God is what gave Shadrach, Meshach and Abednego confidence in the face of death (see Dn 5). Want some homework? Do a Bible study on the attributes or character of God. Learn that He is good, all-powerful, all-knowing, immutable, transcendent, the same yesterday, today and forever. Sooner or later most of us will come to a point when it appears that God has lost control—or interest—in the affairs of our lives. If we try to make sense of God based solely on what we see around us, we will be disappointed. That's when it helps to have a clear view of who God really is. Then we can choose to interpret the things we don't understand in light of the things we do understand. Just for starters, consider this: "One thing God has spoken, two things have I heard: that you, O God, are *strong*, and that you, O Lord, are *loving*" (Ps 62:11-12, emphasis added).

Second, when God *doesn't*, we should view His response in the light of what He says about us in His Word. The truest thing about you and me is what God says about us! God never acts contrary to His Word. Consider these:

- We have been chosen in Christ from before the foundation of the world, and we are predestined to be adopted as sons (Eph 1:4-5).
- We are indwelt by Jesus Christ who is our hope of glory (Col 1:27).
- Nothing can separate us from the love of God (Rom 8:35-39).
- We have been raised from spiritual death to sit together with Christ in the heavenly places (Eph 2:1-6).

Thinking on these truths will help develop in us a deep confidence in God so that when we face life's trials and uncertainties we are able to say, "God, I don't understand what is going on, but I know I matter to You, that You love me unconditionally and are committed to maturing me."

Third, when God *doesn't*, we should trust life's uncertainties to His sovereign plan. Listen to what trust sounds like: "Naked I came from my mother's womb, and naked I will depart. The Lord gave and the Lord has taken away; may the name of the Lord be praised" (Jb 1:21). When Job's wife recommended that he curse God and die, he answered, "Shall we accept good from God, and not trouble?" (Jb 2:10). Trust ranks at the top of God's priorities for us. He wants to be our Provider, Protector, Redeemer, Healer and Supplier of every good and perfect gift. He wants us to come to the end of our resources so that we will depend on His! When you feel like crying out, "Where is God?" you can rest in His promise: "The Lord is close to the brokenhearted and saves those who are crushed in spirit" (Ps 34:18).

One Sunday in Bible school the teacher asked Bobby, "Where is God?" Bobby sat there motionless, not knowing what to say. The teacher asked again, "Where is God?" Bobby ran out of the room to his younger brother and said, "God's *missing*, and they're blaming it on us!" God is not missing. He knows. He cares. True comfort doesn't come from knowing *why*, it comes from knowing God and trusting Him.

Because of this confidence, we, too, can join the chorus of the redeemed and say: "Therefore we do not lose heart. Though outwardly we are wasting away, yet inwardly we are being renewed day by day. For our light and momentary troubles are achieving for us an eternal glory that far outweighs them all. So we fix our eyes not on what is seen, but on what is unseen. For what is seen in temporary, but what is unseen is eternal" (2 Cor 4:16-18).

John Chrysostom was one of the great church fathers. He lived in the fourth century. As a very young Christian he was brought before the emperor, who said that if he would not give up Christ, he would be banished from the country. Chrysostom said, "You cannot, for the whole world is my Father's land. You can't banish me." The emperor said, "Then I will take away all your property." "You cannot. My treasures are in heaven," was his reply. "Then I'll take you to a place where there is not a friend to speak to." Chrysostom replied, "You cannot. I have a friend who is closer than a brother. I shall have Jesus Christ forever." Then the emperor finally threatened, "Then I'll take away your life!" The answer came, "You cannot. My life is hid in God with Christ." And the emperor said, "What do you do with a man like that?"

Lord, grow our understanding of your unchanging character. Grow our ability to trust even when things don't make sense.

**For Group Discussion:**

1. Discuss the comment, "God needs no defense ... but Christians often need an explanation."

2. Share a time in your life when you experienced a *bruise on the soul.*

**Personal Application:**

1. Read and reread the Scripture texts that help us understand how God sees us.

2. Have you stopped asking, "Why?" and started to ask, "How?" and "To what end?"

3. Take the challenge to do a Bible study of the character of God. Here are some places to begin:
   • Deuteronomy 6:4
   • 2 Samuel 22:2
   • Psalm 9:9
   • Psalm 23:1
   • Psalm 27:1
   • Psalm 100:3
   • 2 Corinthians 3:17
   • 2 Thessalonians 3:3
   • Hebrews 13:6

**Just For the Caregiver**

When trying to figure out the reason your loved one is suffering, we sometimes get more frustrated and angry. Take this day to *not focus* on your unanswered questions. Instead, make it a day of trust and thankfulness. *What can you find in your present circumstances to be grateful about?* It could be something as simple as, "At least I have the strength to care for him today," or "My Easter lily is still blooming."

# SEVEN

## Staying Close

**Pamala:** When tragedy strikes a family member it effects everyone involved in some way. In our case a spouse and a father is slowly being taken from us by a degenerative brain disease. Tragedy *will* challenge the strength of a family, proving the statement, "That which does not kill us will make us stronger." Fortunately for our family, the latter has happened. We are stronger as individuals and as a family unit. We made the decision to work together through our tragedy as best we could and to remain close, avoiding the tendency to attack one another.

We have known for six years now that Richard will die and, unless God intervenes, it will be a difficult death. During these six years our family has gone through many changes. For one, we were forced to redefine our family's persona. It was not easy to do and, quite honestly, made all of us nervous. Especially me.

Since Richard's illness is neurological, he suffers from severe mood swings and at times drifts in and out of what we call "fog." His behavior would change, and this caused difficulty for all of us. We found it crucial to direct our fears and frustrations toward something other than Richard. After all, he could not help alter his behavior. It was *the illness,* not Richard causing the disturbance and conflict. Richard and I began referring to the illness as the third person in our marriage. As you can imagine, having a third person involved in a marriage causes a lot of stress.

Unlike a typical third person, though, the disease was always there, refusing to leave us. Denying its existence only caused more frustration; we had to acknowledge its presence. Once we validated the third person, we found it easier to direct the irritation toward it rather than toward each other. It was the disease that took away harmony in our home, the job Richard loved so much and his freedom. Labeling the invader as a third person helped Richard as well as the family to handle our sorrow and loss.

We are past the initial fear and panic the disease has brought to our family. But there is the growing sense of uncertainty for each of us. It is the not knowing what is coming next that continues to wear away at the fabric of our family. Will the next door be the doorway to death, or will it merely open to another passageway of suffering? Nothing is for sure, except that one day the final door of this journey will open and it will lead Richard into the very presence of God. When this happens, all that has taken place in this life will melt away from his memory, or at least it won't cause him any more pain. Richard will then experience ultimate healing in the presence of God. God will comfort our family's loneliness with this confidence. We will face new and different challenges, but this one will be over. Until then we will care for one another, support Richard and depend on God daily for the ability to do all of this with love, and hopefully, no regrets.

Our family has become better at depending on God for strength, provision, wisdom and peace than we ever thought possible. However, along with our dependency, God also wants us to carry our share of the load and not bail out on the responsibilities we face. God will not do for us things we can and should do for ourselves. When things are within our power to accomplish, we should do them. God is not in the habit of indulging His children. His desire is to grow us stronger through each new challenge. I personally have said to Him on many occasions, "I think I am strong enough now; would you just take over?" I know to develop strength and endurance I must be willing to bear my part.

*Life can be compared to a gymnasium.* While we are here on earth everyone is required to spend time working out, all for the purpose of building strength for new challenges that come our way. Building on this metaphor, I would like to recommend a few things I have found helpful to pack in your *gym* bag.

## Acceptance

First, you will have to see your marriage or your family in a different light. Some things can never be the same. There is a sense of powerlessness of neither being able to go backward to the way things used to be, or go forward so you can move on. *It is necessary to face the reality of being in this place for a while and figuring out life right here.* Accepting this reality seems to be the first step in keeping a family healthy during ongoing illness and suffering.

I was resisting this until I had a "moment of reality" with Richard one evening. I had spent most of the week crying and grieving over our loss. I wanted to go back and get my life, give Richard back his life, give the kids their dad and the grandkids their Poppy Richard. As I sat crying with tears pouring down my face, I asked Richard to come over and sit down by me. (He was watching television at the time.) He reluctantly came over and sat beside me, but never taking his eyes off the television screen. I pulled him close and literally buried my face in his chest and bawled loudly. Then without warning, he pushed me away and said, "Did you remember to pick up my favorite salad dressing today?" Stunned, I wiped my face and quietly answered, "Yes, Hon, I remembered."

That was the night I truly accepted the fact that we were never going back to the way things were and I needed to let go of those dreams. I knew I must accept, if not embrace, where we are now and figure out life from here. I needed to figure out a new way to love Richard. I wrote down some ways that would be better for me and for him.

- Love unconditionally, even though the way that love is expressed may be different than it was before.
- Take his feelings seriously.
- Validate his worth by allowing him to do what he can for himself.
- Find something to appreciate about him daily.
- Give him lots of hugs.
- Have realistic expectations of him.
- Be creative in finding fun things we can still do together.
- Place anger toward the disease and not him.
- Find time to spend with him as a noncaregiver.
- Respect his space and privacy and pride as a man.
- Acknowledge every success—no matter how small.
- Talk about normal stuff, not just the illness.
- Give him plenty of smiles (he loves my smile). In fact, I pray that is the last thing he sees this side of heaven.

Creating this list was helpful for Richard and me. I needed to release my expectations and stop insisting he do what he could no longer do. He did not need to feel the pressure of my unmet needs. I asked God for help in managing my unmet needs for comfort, affection, support and friendship. He is a very creative God. He knows each of us better than we know ourselves. He has given me all I have needed to get through this lonely time: grandchildren to cuddle up with, friends to be close to, children who support me. True, my friends cannot always be available to comfort me, but God is. I have found tremendous intimacy alone with Him on my knees in prayer. On many days, I've found myself longing for that special time with Him, when I know He will comfort me. I believe He will do the same for any man, woman or child. The Bible puts it like this: God will be a Father to the fatherless, a husband to the widow and a parent to the orphan (Ex 22:22; Jas 1:27). I have prayed this prayer for my kids and myself. I encourage you to do the same. God created everything—including your needs—and He can meet them in the most amazing and unique ways for as long as He needs to.

## Honesty

Honesty with family and friends has proven to be the best approach when it comes to being asked how Richard and our family are doing. In general, people are very uncomfortable asking about Richard. Some think it humane to try and make him *less* sick by reporting to others that he is doing "fine." But honesty in times of tragedy is what a family needs.

Richard actually wrote a letter to his close family and friends to help them answer questions related to his health.

Richard also included suggestions in this letter:

> To some of my family and friends it remains unclear as to what is wrong with me. The official diagnosis is fronto-temporal dementia. You can go to www.WebMD.com and search their site and find a number of articles that describe the disease in detail.
>
> I have been asked by some friends, "What should I say when somebody asks, 'How is Richard doing?'" I don't know if it's appropriate for me to offer suggestions in this area, but there has been some confusion and I think it would help if we were on the same page. Here are some things that would be appropriate to say:
>
> 1. Richard's health continues to decline.
> 2. He is living alone so that he can be in a quiet, managed environment.
> 3. He has had to recently give up his driving privileges (this has been really hard).
> 4. Unless God intervenes, he will suffer from all the symptoms associated with dementia.
> 5. Richard agrees with the psalmist: "All the days ordained for me were written in your book before one of them came to be" (Ps 139:16). Richard wants to live as long as God wants him to live—not a day longer nor a day shorter.
> 6. Richard and Pamala have agreed in prayer that when God is finished with Richard's purpose here on earth that He—in His mercy—will take him home.

I don't much care for this "list" approach to correspondence with family and friends, but I want to be as open and transparent as I can about how I am doing and what you can do to help. Someone has said, "Friendship doubles our joy and divides our grief."

Thank you for being my friend,
*Richard*

## A Network of Good Support

**Pamala:** I cannot emphasize enough the necessity of having a network of positive encouragers. (We will cover this idea in even more detail in chapter ten.) These are people who will let you cry as well as allow you to laugh on occasion. You must have this in your gym bag at all times.

We all need someone we can call anytime, day or night. Every family member should avoid isolation. Isolation can lead to depression, and depression is called "the common cold of mental illness." A type of emotional hypothermia takes place as a person gets cold from being alone. In some cases, the person can shut down his or her emotions completely. I have already admitted I was doing this very thing in the beginning. I was definitely moving into a serious state of depression. I had to get people back into my life again. I needed to be emotionally strong so I could help Richard and our family.

Look for a good support network to help you during this lengthy period of suffering. You need friends who will be committed for the long haul. Many will fall by the wayside as the months and years go by. How very blessed we are to have a few faithful ones still with us, calling, coming by, sending a card or planning a day of fun for me. Thank you. You know who you are, and so do we. We will never forget.

To venture into the dark valley of death without a few close friends is tragic. Jean Vanier says it well: "Wounded people who have been broken by suffering and sickness ask for only one thing: a heart that loves and commits itself to them, a heart full of hope for them."[1] I agree. The vast population will not understand what your family is going through. You will not have enough time or energy to explain or defend the whys and hows of the daily pressures and decisions you must make. But having a network of compassionate people who will pray for and support you through this horrific daze is priceless.

### Good Counseling

We have discovered the value of getting the perspective of a Christian counselor. Granted, friends may provide much-needed support, but there is great value in a trained professional. Our close friend Dr. Lance Lee was present in the room with us when Dr. Mastrianni gave Richard his diagnosis. During the following year Dr. Lee wept when we wept and held our hands when we could weep no more. He has visited our family in Oklahoma, and we have his cell phone number on speed dial and his Email address. Many counselors arrange their fees based on your income, so don't assume that you cannot afford this kind of support. Your local Hospice may be another option for support and good counseling.

Galen Lassiter, executive director of Crossroads Hospice of Oklahoma, says it is overwhelming for a family when they realize their loved one will soon be absent from their lives. Fatigue and stress complicate matters further. Hospice has found it is necessary for family members to be able to talk honestly with someone who is not part of the family to sort through the emotions they may be feeling, to solve problems associated with the relationship, or talk about complications of providing patient care. Hospice provides bereavement counselors, social workers, chaplains and nurses.

In addition to providing bereavement counseling for a period of thirteen months after the loss of your loved one, hospice also provides help with "anticipatory" grief. This is grief associated with the incremental losses the family and patient experience even before a death, such as loss of health, independence, dreams, identity, goals and relationships. Get the support you and your family need both during the anticipatory phase of grief, as well as after your loved one is gone.

A letter from the patient's doctor stating that death could be imminent within six months is now the requirement to obtain Hospice service. However, efforts are being made to extend this time period to twelve months. You can look in your local Yellow Pages to contact the nearest Hospice to find out what services might be available for your family.

## A Sense of Humor

You've heard the saying, "Laughter is the best medicine." Our family has found this to be true. As often as you can, laugh together.

Richard was a city slicker from Northern California most of his life. He spent about ten days total in Oklahoma prior to his illness and would list those ten days among his forty worst days ever. He does not care for country music, hates flat land, cannot tolerate humidity and despises fried okra—all words he used to describe Oklahoma. He is amazed at God's sense of humor. Richard said to me, "Oklahoma? I must be dying! If I believed in penance I would swear this is it!" He often tells me not to worry about what I am going to make for dinner; he cannot even recall what he had for lunch. This may seem like crude humor to you, but it makes us laugh about our real life. If you can laugh together as a family it will help you manage very real and difficult challenges taking place in your life.

## Communication

To stay on top of how everyone is doing you must talk and reveal your honest feelings. It's also important to understand that members of your family may have different preferences for and styles of communicating. Sometimes you must provide a nonthreatening atmosphere for this to take place. Our girls always wanted to talk late at night. Apryl would just come right out with what was on her mind; she is still that way. Amy needs to warm up first, feel safe, and then talk. Aaron is different. He only wants to talk about serious stuff on a need-to-know basis.

We learned this about Aaron when he was little and had questions about sex. Aaron started being inquisitive about some sexual matters that his friends had been talking about. During the day he came and asked me his question over and over. I wanted Richard to handle this since I had done the "sex talk" with both the girls. I felt it was only fair for Richard to have his turn! So when Aaron asked me his questions I would simply say, "Aaron, that's a good question, but you need to wait and ask your dad when he gets home tonight." Dad did get home and as he was tucking Aaron into bed that night, sure enough, he asked his dad the same questions he had asked me. Richard gave him enough information to satisfy, but not too much to overwhelm him. Aaron seemed content with his new knowledge. But just as Richard was turning to leave Aaron's room he said, "Hey Dad, you need to explain this stuff to Mom, 'cause she don't know nothin' about sex!" Like I said, only on a need-to-know basis.

Keeping the door of communication open provides opportunities to tell stories like this one and humiliate your kids forever! It also makes it so much easier to deal with tragedy in an honest and healthy way.

It is also important if you are the primary caregiver that you do *not* take onto your own shoulders the role of communicating for everybody, or communicating in a way that protects others from the truth. Richard told the kids about his illness initially, but soon after I pretty much kept them informed about how things were going. However, we soon realized it was far better for him to speak with the kids when he felt up to it. They needed to hear news from him, not me. I had thought I was making it easier; I wanted to protect both Richard and the kids from the stress of the illness. But in doing this, things appeared to be easier for me than they really were and I did not receive the support I needed. The family was also getting disillusioned about what was actually going on. We have found that the more transparent you are with family about what is really happening, the more support you will receive from them.

**Deal With Stuff**

You can deal with stuff now, or deal with stuff later, but stuff must be dealt with. Some people want to put off today what can be dealt with tomorrow, but tomorrow eventually does come. It is a waste of time dreading certain conversations, decisions or actions that must take place. It is best to face them as soon as possible. Nike's "just do it" philosophy is the appropriate way to face any dreaded task.

Be assured that when the family is in an ongoing crisis of a lengthy illness, difficult issues or dysfunctions that have been going on in the marriage or in the family before the illness will surface and become even more obvious. If siblings were having a riff before Dad got sick, the problem will likely escalate. If a couple's relationship was rocky before the illness, there will be even more distance between them now. Stuff does not just go away during the slow motion of lengthy suffering.

To survive and keep the family as emotionally healthy as possible, do not run from the obvious. Talk about it. Be as honest as possible. Call a truce; admit truth to the kids, friends and family. The illness may be a very long haul and you do not want to pack unnecessary baggage for the trip.

A network of supporters, counselors, humor, open communication and dealing with stuff head-on—these are some things we as a family have placed in *our* gym bag. We are presently in very good shape, but we know we have a ways to go. It is our desire to remain close as a family and to complete this lengthy workout in better condition than when we began. In spite of all the difficulties, we have discovered we have become more compassionate, merciful, long-suffering, deeper, wiser, and definitely closer to each other and God.

### Advice For the One Who Is Ill

**Richard:** From my perspective, I would like to offer to the person who is ill the following suggestions for your own gym bag. You will want to make your contribution to keeping your family close too.

1. *Don't cling.* Give the other person the space he or she needs. Both of you have your own special set of needs. I know as the sick person I have had to struggle not to cling to Pamala. I leaned on her too much for emotional support in the past, so it was only natural that I would follow the same pattern. Clinging can lead to suffocating the other person, thus driving them away from you.

2. *Do thank your caregivers for their time.* It is so easy to want more time, more attention, more emotional support and more sympathy. But the person we love the most is only capable of giving so much. Rather than being cranky and cantankerous, learn to thank your loved one for taking the time to help you or visit you. Showing your genuine appreciation will go a long way in keeping your relationship close.

3. *Do let them know what you need.* Playing hide-and-seek will wring the joy out of any relationship. Let your loved one know what you need from them. Even if they are unable to meet the need, perhaps they know of a resource that can address it. Staying close requires that there is openness. Staying close is a two-way street.

4. *Do ask them if there is anything you can do for them.* That may seem unlikely in some circumstances, but you may be surprised that—even with your limitations—you can provide a valuable service to your loved one. It may catch them off guard, but I can assure you they will appreciate the fact that you are thinking of them and their needs.

5. *Do ask them how you can pray for them.* It's a simple question, but it can provide a huge emotional lift to someone who is carrying a heavy load. Of course, it should go without saying, you should take notes and then pray for them and their specific needs. They suffer, too. And who better than you can understand what they are going through?

6. *Do ask them to be open and honest with you.* It is the tendency of the caregiver to want to protect the sufferer. I suppose there are exceptions to this suggestion, but we should let our loved one know that we want them to be open and honest with us about anything concerning our medical condition, financial matters and the like. Most days I feel like the bent wheel on a shopping cart but I do want to do what I can. I don't want to be kept in the dark.

7. *Do ask them, "Is there anything you want to say to me?"* Pamala and I have had the practice of asking one another—often at unexpected moments—"Is there anything you want to say to me?" You might think that's a loaded question but it opens the door for the other person to give expression to something they may have been thinking about but were waiting for the right time to say it. Staying close demands that we are "speak-

ing the truth in love" (Eph 4:15). You may need to brace yourself, but I would rather experience an open relationship than just the outward appearance, wouldn't you?

8. *Do work to make your time together quality time.* I know our circumstances vary, but when we spend time with our loved one we need to do our best to get in a frame of mind to enjoy and celebrate our time together. Often before family gatherings I whisper a prayer and ask God to give me a sense of anticipation and an attitude that will contribute to an enjoyable time. It is easy to get sour. It is easy to think about ourselves above others. Don't waste the time you have by pouting.

9. *Do reflect on your actions and activities.* This subject is dealt with more completely in chapter twelve, but reflecting on our activities in a journal is one key in keeping our lives tracking in the right direction. Small course corrections are easier to make than major overhauls.

10. *Do ask God for an attitude of gratitude.* Our disposition is so important in life. While we have no control over our circumstances, we do have control over our attitude. God is ready to help us grow an attitude of gratitude. My aim has been, "Be joyful in hope, patient in affliction, and faithful in prayer" (Rom 12:12).

## For Group Discussion:
1. Do you find yourself living with a "third person"? If you are comfortable, explain the circumstances to the group.
2. Pamala recommends that acceptance of the facts as they

are should be the first item to put in your "gym bag." Have you really come to terms with your trials and the true nature of them?

3. Richard took the initiative and gave suggestions to his close friends and family about how to answer questions people had about his condition. Would you feel comfortable taking such action? Why or why not?

**For Personal Application:**

1. In addition to supportive friends, we may need the assistance of professional Christian counselors. Is this an action step that you need to take?

2. Staying close requires openness and communication. What have you been putting off? When do you plan to do something about it?

3. From the suggestions that Pamala and Richard have offered, which items need to find their way into your gym bag?

**Just For the Caregiver**

In this chapter Pamala gives a list of loving ways to demonstrate genuine affection to your loved one. From the list of thirteen ways she listed, choose one or two you can apply this week in the life of your loved one. Give them a word of encouragement, no matter how small.

Also for you, the caregiver, to receive adequate help and support you must communicate honestly about the progress of the illness from time to time. One way you can help your family and friends to stay in touch with your needs is to provide information. The key here is to give important and helpful information without a lot of effort on your part. You may want to compile and set up an Email address box that contains the Email addresses of all your close friends and family members. You can type a note once every two weeks; just hit the "send" button and you have informed many people about how they can pray and support you intelligently. Richard has always preferred the use of letters (along with Email).

Take some time this week to begin a first draft (on paper) of a note you can send as an Email when the information reads like you want it to read. And if you don't have Email, there is always snail mail! You can also set up a regular time to update close family members, like a once-a-week call (or even once a month). Even if they do not like what they hear, they need to know how it really is. If you are questioned about how you are handling matters, you can always answer those questions by simply inviting them to come and spend time with your loved one while you take a day off!

EIGHT

## The God of All Comfort

**Richard:** I like it when the road ahead is smooth and the wind is to my back. Don't you? The highway close to my house is presently under construction. Orange cones, traffic, dump trucks and dirt. Lots of dirt. If Pamala is driving through a construction zone, she will say something like, "Just think of how nice it will be when the work is done!" or "Won't it be nice when the new lane is opened up?" But just the thought of a construction zone makes me wonder if I really need to go anywhere or not. Life is a lot like that.

I prefer the kind of life-signs that read, *Smooth Roads Ahead, Children All Walking With God,* or *Perfect Health.* But sooner or later we all come upon construction zones, and signs like *Merger Ahead, Expect Delays,* or *Detour* begin to appear. Know what I mean?

So far I have come across five distinct construction zones along the road of my illness, and so far God has met me at every "Why?" in the road. But before I share my life's experiences with construction zones, let me offer the glimpse of God's character that is so important to consider.

It is God's nature to comfort His children. Listen to these words: "Praise be to the God and Father of our Lord Jesus Christ, the Father of compassion and *the God of all comfort,* who comforts us in all our troubles, so that we can comfort those in any trouble with the comfort we ourselves have received from God. For just as the sufferings of Christ flow over into our lives, so also through Christ our comfort overflows" (2 Cor 1:3-5, emphasis added).

Life's constructions zones do not surprise God. I have learned that the providence of God paves the way to a deep belief in God's ability to help us navigate life's potholes. The word *providence* comes from two Latin words. The prefix *pro* indicates "before" or "in front of." The root comes from the Latin *videre*, which means "to see." Put together we have a word that means "to see beforehand." But the doctrine of providence goes much beyond this brief definition.

First, providence refers to God's *provision* for His people. While we all labor to make provision for our families, Jesus taught us not to worry about what we would eat, drink or wear. Our worry and anxiety are to be assuaged by our confidence in the provision of God for His people.

Providence also encompasses the idea of God's *paternal care* for His children. This means God is involved in human affairs. He is not a God who acted in Creation and since then stands aloof and uninvolved in human history. It is only as we learn to trust God that we are able to experience His comfort.

Before I identify my experience with life's construction zones, I encourage you to keep this attribute of God in mind, and I offer this disclaimer: what follows is not suited for a Hallmark greeting card. I didn't read this somewhere and decide to pass it along to you. I am presently in a construction zone and I have spent some time "between the orange cones." I am offering a firsthand view from here.

**Construction Zone #1:** *Shame Ahead*

A sense of shame and condemnation can come from a number of sources. It can come from the realization that, apart from Christ, the wrath of God abides on us (Jn 3:18). We can sense condemnation or shame when we are thrown to the mat by a besetting sin (Heb 12:1). But shame also comes at those times when we feel inadequate, when we fail to get a promotion, when we are being cut from the team. And shame can come directly from the accuser of our brothers, Satan himself. "Now have come the salvation and the power and the kingdom of our God, and the authority of his Christ. For the accuser of our brothers, who accuses them [Christians] before our God day and night, has been hurled down" (Rv 12:10). Satan busies himself—*day and night*—hurling accusations with the intent to cause us shame. But God's comfort can be found in this declaration: "Therefore, there is now no condemnation for those who are in Christ Jesus" (Rom 8:1).

In his book, *Will Daylight Come?*, Robert Heffler pens this moving illustration:

> There was a little boy visiting his grandparents on their farm. He was given a slingshot to play with out in the woods where he practiced but could never hit the target. Becoming discouraged, he headed back to lunch. As he was walking along he saw Grandma's pet duck, and impulsively, he let fly, hit the duck square in the head, and killed it. He was shocked and grieved. In a panic, he hid the dead duck in the woodpile ... only to discover his sister watching. Sally had seen it all, but she said nothing.
>
> After lunch that day, Grandma said, "Sally, let's wash

the dishes." But Sally said, "Grandma, Johnny told me he wanted to help in the kitchen today, *didn't you Johnny?*" And then she whispered to him, "Remember the duck?"

So Johnny did the dishes.

Later, Grandpa asked if the children wanted to go fishing and Grandma said, "I'm sorry but I need Sally to help make supper." But Sally smiled and said, "Well that's all right because Johnny told me he wanted to help." And she whispered again, "Remember the duck?" So Sally went fishing and Johnny stayed home.

After several days of Johnny doing both his chores and Sally's, he finally couldn't stand it any longer. He came to Grandma and confessed that he had killed the duck. She knelt down, gave him a hug, and said, "Sweetheart, I know. You see, I was standing at the window and I saw the whole thing. But because I love you, I forgave you. I was just wondering how long you would let Sally make a slave of you."[1]

I don't know what "ducks" are in your past. I don't know what one sin the accuser keeps throwing up in your face. But Jesus Christ was standing at the window and saw the whole thing. He has forgiven you through His work on the cross. He is wondering how long you and I will let the accuser make a slave out of us. Take comfort in His forgiveness.

**Construction Zone #2:** *Desert Experiences*

Sand. Lots of sand. For forty years that thought must have gone through Moses' mind. Moses got ahead of God and had to wait forty years for his number to be called again. I am not suggesting this is the "norm," but we all have desert experiences. Sometimes, our desert experiences are the result of our own doing (as in the case of Moses) and, other times, they are for no apparent reason (as in the case of Job).

At the end of forty long years, Moses reminded God's people of an important lesson learned in the desert.

> *Remember how the Lord your God led you all the way in the desert these forty years, to humble you and to test you in order to know what was in your heart, whether or not you would keep his commands. He humbled you, causing you to hunger and then feeding you with manna, which neither you nor your fathers had known, to teach you that man does not live on bread alone but on every word that comes from the mouth of the Lord.*
>
> DEUTERONOMY 8:2-3

In the case of the children of Israel, God *humbled* them and He *caused* them to go hungry. Sound strange? It shouldn't. Just as God knew what was in *their* hearts, so God knows what is in *ours.* He wants us to know. And so the desert experiences come.

No doubt the Sinai desert seemed God-forsaken, but God has never forsaken—nor will he ever forsake—His kids. He was the water that gushed from the rock. He sent a banquet (quail and manna). He made a fashion statement (shoes that lasted forty years!). But when you are in a desert experience, it can seem like God is a million miles away.

As tough as it may seem, the key question to ask in a desert experience is not "Why?" but "What?" Take comfort that God has your best interest at heart.

## Construction Zone #3: *Friendly Fire*

Strange term, *friendly fire*. But that's what they called it as we—for the first time and as a nation—watched the war in Vietnam from our living rooms. Friendly fire was death by accident. It was death at the hands of your allies. Imagine the grief a mother felt as she read the telegram and learned that her son had been killed by his own troops—by friendly fire. Sent twelve thousand miles from home and killed by friends.

In contrast, I use the term more loosely. Few things in life wound us like friendly fire: reckless words, false accusations, jealous remarks and spiteful comments. With a few short sentences, a "friend" can tear down a reputation it took a lifetime to build. It seems that, the further toward the front you move in leadership, the more likely friendly fire is to come upon you. I have sat dazed, wondering how God could possibly work friendly fire for the good of those who love Him. Frankly, this is one construction zone I don't understand. But God has taught me that the urge to retaliate or the temptation to take my marbles and go home are both wrong responses to friendly fire.

## Construction Zone #4: *Fatigue*

I have flirted with fatigue most of my life. Maybe it is my need to achieve, or whatever, but I am all too familiar with the subject. I have learned that fatigue comes in a variety of forms. I have gotten more acquainted with *physical* fatigue as I have grown older. But even young men and women can struggle with *spiritual* and *emotional* fatigue.

Elijah was so worn out he wanted to die (1 Kgs 19:1-4). The prophet Isaiah also knew we could all come face-to-face with fatigue at one time or another. He reminds us:

*Do you not know? Have you not heard? The Lord is the ever-lasting God, the Creator of the ends of the earth. He will not grow tired or weary, and his understanding no one can fathom. He gives strength to the weary and increases the power of the weak. Even youths grow tired and weary, and young men stumble and fall; but those who hope in the Lord will renew their strength. They will soar on wings like eagles; they will run and not grow weary, they will walk and not be faint.*

ISAIAH 40:28-31

As in the case of Elijah, God uses fatigue to get our attention and to remind us that He is the Source of our strength. God instructed Elijah to rest and to eat something. But God had more in mind for Elijah than a few days of vacation in Horeb. While Elijah was safe at the entrance of a cave, God sent a powerful wind that tore the mountains, but God was not in the wind. He sent an earthquake, but God was not in the earthquake. Then came a fire, but God was not in the fire. And then God came. He came in a gentle whisper. I have at least one thing in common with the great prophet—neither of us "do" quietness very well. For those of us who prefer the wind and fire, God knows what we need. Sooner or later, the fatigued must heed God's invitation to "Be still, and know that I am God" (Ps 46:10). Take comfort that God stands beside you.

**Construction Zone #5:** *The Unknown*
Few things paralyze us like the unknown. And when it comes to life, there are plenty of unknowns. Living in the face of the unknown can lead to a bad case of the "What Ifs?" Then anxiety can set in and contaminate our mind and heart, and we

grind to a halt. Solomon was right: "An anxious heart weighs a man down" (Prv 12:25).

In the Bible we have more accounts of God greeting people at their point of fear than at any other life circumstance. God's "Fear not" greeted the likes of Abram, Hagar, Moses, Joshua, Zacharias, Joseph and Mary, to name only a few. And the reason God gives the command that we should not fear is the promise of His own presence. "So do not fear, for I am with you" (Is 41:10). God is not the author of fear. "For God did not give us a spirit of timidity, but a spirit of power, of love and of self-discipline" (2 Tm 1:7).

However, the *knowledge* of God's pledge to be ever-present does not keep us from *feeling* life's fears. We face new circumstances, new trials and new construction zones. I remember one specific time when I felt the grip of fear tighten around my neck. I was reluctant to share my feelings with anyone because I knew some of my fears were nothing but unfounded paranoia. So while at my favorite coffee shop, I tore a sheet of paper out of my binder and, at the top, I wrote: "FEARS—Real or Otherwise." I was determined to list my fears. Seeing them on paper helped me get a handle on them. Then I went to God's Word and searched for His promises as they related directly to my fears. (You can conduct the same kind of search with a concordance or Bible software program.) On this specific occasion, God especially used Psalm 91 to touch me at my greatest point of need.

Psalm 91 begins with a declaration of the greatness of God: "He who dwells in the shelter of the Most High will rest in the shadow of the Almighty." When I was a kid, my playmates and I would get into shouting matches with one another. When things would get tense, our final resort would be to say, "Oh yeah? Well, my brother is bigger than your brother!" The only problem was, I didn't *have* a brother! We took courage and comfort in the fact that we knew somebody who was bigger and stronger. The words "the *shadow* of the Almighty" paint the picture of God's bigness and strength. That is enough to put my fears in perspective.

In verses 3-8, various calamities are described but our fears are addressed with this promise: "For he will command his angels concerning you to guard you in all your ways; they will lift you up in their hands, so that you will not strike your foot against a stone" (vv. 11-12). Does God promise to take away any and all potential episodes of fear? No. Does He promise a life of ease and isolation from the struggles of life? Hardly. But God does promise that, when we call upon him, "I will answer him; I will be with him in trouble, I will deliver him and honor him" (v. 15). Take comfort that God's angelic hosts are at His disposal to guard His children.

### More Construction Zones

**Pamala:** The construction zone our family is currently held up in is not a comfortable one. We are in the wait mode. We can't go backward to when Richard was well, and we can't move forward beyond his illness either. It is a difficult place to be.

But I was reminded recently that if I were to look around at the suffering of others I just might decide to choose the heartache we have. It's like the story of the man who was complaining to God about the cross he was called to carry here on earth. God asked him if he wanted to choose another. The man was thrilled at the opportunity to exchange his wearisome cross for another easier one. He gladly turns in his cross to God, and is then shown to the "cross room" to choose another. After looking around the room at the enormous, hideous looking crosses, he sees a tiny one leaning against the wall. He asks God, "Can I have the one over there, against the wall?" God says, "Well sure, but it's the one you just returned to me."

The following are stories of other fellow sufferers. Perhaps after reading about the cross each of them carries you will say, "No thank you, I'll keep the one I have."

**Deeper Truths**

**Written by Kimbra's little sister, now a thirty-six–year-old woman:** I used to think the abbreviation B.C. and A.D. could only be "Before Christ" and "After His death." However, after my sixteen-year-old sister was diagnosed with terminal cancer, those letters took on a whole new meaning. I started to compare everything to "before cancer" and "after her death." Life "before" meant having a "normal" family who loved one another, went to church and had money to spend on all of our needs and most of our wants. You see, cancer brought trials into our lives that never existed "B.C."

At the age of fourteen I suddenly became aware of our mounting medical bills, parents who were absent more than present, and a sister struggling with hair loss, sleepless nights and the thought of dying at a young age.

I struggled with comparing my life to my friends. Their parents weren't hundreds of miles away visiting different hospitals. They didn't work at a young age to help make ends meet. And they certainly didn't have to watch their loved one deteriorate before their eyes! God was no stranger to my hidden anger. Little did I know that what I would experience through my sister's battle would stay with me for the rest of my life.

I watched my parents develop a deeper hunger for God and His Word. They would put Bible verses on my sister's walls and ceiling that would remind her of God's love for her and His healing power. I matured from a selfish teenager into someone who truly saw that "all of our lives are but a vapor!" I watched as people brought groceries to our door and held prayer meetings on our behalf. But only Christ could sustain us 24/7!

The Lord spoke to me sometimes in my spirit and sometimes in those few intimate moments, where time seemed to stand still. One memory stands out the most. One evening about a month before Kim's death, my mom woke me about 3:00 A.M. She wanted to know if I could rub my sister's arms and legs and pray over her for a while. You see, the cancer had spread to her bones and elsewhere at a rapid rate and the morphine had no effect anymore. My parents were exhausted and I agreed to take a turn. As I sat beside her bed I felt so helpless. I slowly started to speak a few Bible verses over her (I only knew a few back then). As I prayed, I asked God to turn her screams of pain into a blanket of peace and rest that would hover for the night. After a few minutes I realized God had answered and she slept the rest of the night.

On June 27, 1968, Kim took her last breath, but not before she said these words: "Family together" and "Jesus."

Does cancer hurt? Yes. But the A.D. (after her death) has only revealed deeper truths about God's unfailing love. As I said earlier, B.C. (before cancer) meant we had a normal family. We loved each other, went to church and had no financial worries. But the Lord replaced all of that with a revelation of Himself and an even deeper love within our family, as well as spiritual riches beyond compare.

## When Alzheimer's Strikes

**Written by seventy-seven-year-old Mabel:** Alzheimer's is a very cruel disease. It is hard for the caregivers and the family to see such a change in the one they love. My husband was the one I depended on to remember all the dates, times and years that important things happened. I first knew something was really wrong when one day on the way home he asked me which way to turn. On another occasion he was driving in the passing lane on the turnpike and I told him he should get into his own lane. He turned on the signal to change lanes, but didn't turn it off. After a while I told him to turn off the signal and he said, "I can't turn off the signal and drive at the same time."

He has gone from over 200 pounds to 135. He has gone back to being a child. He can't dress himself, bathe, shave or do the things he used to do. He used to be so neat and clean; now he wears Depends and can't control his bladder and a lot of times his bowels.

The doctor tells me I'm lucky he has such a sweet disposition. He wants me right alongside him most of the time. He still tells me how much he loves me. Once he said, "My head feels so crazy."

He can't get out of bed by himself any longer. I help him at night when he says he has to go to the bathroom. But when he gets there he asks, "What do you want me to do?" He can't carry on a conversation or tell me what he wants. He forgets what he is trying to say. He lives in his own little world. He goes all through the house changing things or playing with coins. He plays for hours just picking up coins and moving them around.

We can see him losing ground about every week. We just take it a day at a time and give him our love and care.

### Changed in an Instant

**By Pamala, as told to her by George and Bobbie:** George is a twenty-six-year-old man, married with two children. Until July 4th, 2002, his life looked pretty good. He had a steady job, a home and a wife, Bobbie, who was a stay-at-home mom and a part-time college student. "But things changed in an instant when a Roman candle went off and hit me directly in the right eye," George says. "In an instant all of our lives changed." Listen as George describes the changes in his own words:

- I was instantly blind in one eye.
- I lost my job and due to an oversight I was not covered by insurance.
- We lost our home.
- Bobbie had to quit school and began working at a local bakery making $7.50 an hour to buy necessities like food and medicine, while I stayed home with the boys.
- I was depressed and felt worthless. I was used to taking care of everyone, not others taking care of me.
- We had to file for bankruptcy.
- We were forced to move in with Bobbie's grandmother.
- I went from being a good-looking man to a man who was burned and scarred.

"My self esteem was so low; no one wanted to look at me. I didn't think I would make it, but through the help of neighbors and people from our church I have survived. These people came through when we needed help. I can honestly say the accident forced me to make some needed changes in my life. I am now back in school and I have a dream of becoming a high school coach someday. We still struggle financially, but we are on our way out of this difficultly and on to a better place. The way has not been easy. But I have a new trust in God as He has held our family in His arms many times. I have been encouraged by His love for me, even when others thought me unlovely. I completely trust Him with whatever is ahead. I know that I have been changed forever by a moment of carelessness, but God has used it to bring about good in our lives and in the lives of others."

## Reflections on Losing a Brother

**Written by Ken's grown sister:** I was a junior in high school when I found out my brother Ken had cancer. I remember feeling shock and disbelief and thinking, "People who are eighteen don't get cancer." It seemed so unfair.

The next few years were a blur filled with tears, fear, denial and anger. I had trouble feeling happy. I felt guilty about doing anything positive, knowing that the rest of my family was home fighting for life and hope. I left for college; everyone— including Ken—said I should go, but a part of me just wanted to stay home and help.

After I left, things got worse—much worse—but no one told me the truth. I guess they did not want me to quit school and they didn't want to scare me. They, especially Mom, probably didn't want us to lose our faith, so we never really talked ... never.

That for me then was one of the hardest, most difficult, dichotomies of the Christian walk, and it still is. How does one walk in the shadow of possible or certain physical death while staying in complete faith for healing? How does one stay faith-filled, yet not abandon your humanity and your need to say what you need to say through it all?

We were truly warriors of the faith in the very best way we knew how. We did believe—*I* did believe—that God would, did, and *had* healed Ken completely. We were merely waiting to see it be manifested in the natural. I had much, Much, MUCH more faith than a grain of mustard seed, yet Ken left us to meet the Lord. And I never got to say the hundreds of things I *ached* to say:

- I love you and I'll miss you!
- I'm sorry for ... all the sister stuff.
- I'm sorry for the pain you feel.
- Are you afraid to die?
- What can I say/do/sing to make you feel better?
- I will see you again soon.
- Jesus will meet you and you will not be alone.
- You are brave ... you have been *very* brave.
- Can I cry with you and hold you?

After losing my brother here on earth I couldn't stop thinking about him. The good and the painful memories were con-stantly with me. Years later I felt guilty if I didn't think about him. I would force myself to think about him as if to honor his life. But what I used to see as a "hole" in our family I now see as heaven's addition. The knowledge of his joy in heaven over-shadows my selfish desire to have him here.

## Losing a Child

**Ray:** In her freshman year, my fourteen-year-old daughter, Joyce, suffered a neck and back injury. The neck injury got the most attention at the time and she wore a brace for a while. But it was the back injury that continued to give her problems. A couple of months passed and she experienced even greater difficulty with her back. Nothing helped. So her chiropractor decided we should call in a neurologist. After they did some scans they discovered that Joyce had a tumor in her back that was pressing on her spinal column and sciatic nerve. They flew my wife and Joyce to Minneapolis by air ambulance right away. Then my wife told me it was serious stuff and I flew to join them.

We sat around a conference table with three or four doctors and specialists. The tests showed she had a rare cancer called Ewing's sarcoma and that it was terminal. There were no known survivors of Ewing's and they could only give her a couple of years of quality life if she started chemotherapy right away. Time stood still. Then I excused myself, went to the rest room and threw up.

Joyce was fun and vibrant. Pretty. Tall, but graceful. She had won the Wolf Man Jack dance contest at the local teen hangout. Wolf Man had come all the way from California to our little town and he had personally chosen Joyce the winner and had given her the trophy. Joyce loved dancing—even with her dad. She was becoming a fine basketball player and at 5'10" and growing, the coaches had their eyes on her. She loved the

Lord and was excited about helping to manage a new teenage nightclub in town, "The Turning Point."

The chemotherapy was horrendous. It was powerful poison designed to kill off the weaker cancer cells. It would tear up her stomach and cause her whole body to wrench and convulse as she vomited over and over and over. It is heartbreaking for parents to see chemo ... sickness ... weakness ... feeling better ... cancer cells dying ... a couple of weeks of normalcy ... cancer flares up ... sickness ... weakness ... feeling better. And she lost her long beautiful hair.

Then one day the doctors said there was nothing else they could do. We brought Joyce home from our final trip to Minneapolis. And we were alone with God. It's not the worst place to be. But Joyce grew worse and was bedridden. The cancer had spread. She would cry out day and night from the pain. Nothing prescribed seemed to stop it.

All the while Joyce was listening to tapes of God's Word and praying. She was also studying her schoolwork. The school provided a private tutor and Kim studied. She studied hard, constantly interrupted by pain. But she did it. She graduated from Aberdeen Central High and couldn't wait to see the graduation ceremonies live on television. She waited for her name to be read with the others ... and she waited ... and waited, but it never came. They had forgotten her. Her spirit slumped. Again she suffered the other kind of pain that comes from being forgotten or ignored. Her closest friends stopped coming over and her boyfriend joined the Air Force just because he couldn't stand to see her suffer anymore. He resigned from the Air Force right after her death.

Joyce passed away just a couple of weeks after graduating

from high school. Family and intimate friends surrounded her as she breathed her last breath on earth and then took her first full breath of heaven ... and took her first painless step toward Jesus.

It hurts to lose a child. It leaves an empty place. God fills it after a while. Not all the way, but it becomes manageable and then it becomes a good memory. But when you are a Christian and you know where she is, Whom she is with and that you will see her again—well, it's OK.

There is so much more that could be written. Three years is a long time for a young girl to suffer, and her family with her. But the years since have more than made up for it. The end result was victory in other areas of our lives. We have been able to minister to others in the same circumstances and every one of us knows and serves the Lord in a new and excited way.

**Richard:** One thing is certain; there are more construction zones ahead for all of us. Do whatever you need to do to remind yourself of the promises of God. His Word is a reflection of His character. And it is in God's character to comfort His children. Remember His pledge: "'For I know the plans I have for you,' declares the Lord, 'plans to prosper you and not to harm you, plans to give you hope and a future. Then you will call upon me and come and pray to me, and I will listen to you. You will seek me and find me when you seek me with all your heart'" (Jer 29:11-13).

**Group Discussion:**
1. Which construction zone are you most familiar with?
2. Have you identified comfort points of your own? Can you share them?

3. How would you counsel someone who is facing God's silence?

**Personal Application:**
1. Take the time to read through Psalm 91 and to journal your thoughts.
2. Identify three comfort points of your own. Write them on 3x5 cards and carry them with you this week as a reminder of God's promises. Better yet, post them as a screensaver on your computer at home or work.
3. Reflecting on your most recent construction zone, what key thoughts should you write down for future reference?

**Just For the Caregiver**
As a caregiver we can get bogged down with our "cross to bear." One of the best ways for me to get over having a Pamala Pity Party is to remind myself of the sufferings of others. Who do you know that also has a burden they are called to carry? Do something thoughtful for them today. Take your mind off yourself and bless someone with a card, a call or maybe a movie. Reflect on this passage taken from The Message:

> *All praise to the God and Father of our Master, Jesus the Messiah! Father of all mercy! God of all healing counsel! He comes alongside us when we go through hard times, and before you know it, he brings us alongside someone else who is going through hard times so that we can be there for that person just as God was there for us.*

> 2 CORINTHIANS 1:3-4, THE MESSAGE

**Part III**

**SURVIVAL SKILLS**

# NINE

## The Importance of Family and Friends

**Richard:** I mentioned earlier in the book that "friendship doubles our joy and divides our grief." I can vouch for that. However, my experiences with friends during my time of loss have been mixed at best.

I am not the easiest guy to get to know. I think I am friendly, but I don't make friends easily. I don't just "share my heart" with every passerby. What I'm trying to say is that I only have a few very close friends, but they mean the world to me.

When my illness and economic reasons forced us to move to a different state, it separated me from the few close friends I had. I wasn't prepared for the kind of effect the move would have on my relationships. We promised to keep in touch. A few even visited us after we moved. But over time the phone calls became less frequent and the Emails slowed to a crawl. The harsh reality is that my friends are getting on with their lives. I also feel disadvantaged because my closest friends now live in different states. One is in Ohio, another in Florida, and others in California. I remember and hold on to our relationships as they once were, but many of them have moved ahead with new friends. I do have nearby friends from my last place of ministry, but I also cherish my friends from years past. I feel like a kid on Christmas morning when I hear the voice of one of my dear friends. I have drawn the most comfort from those I have known the longest.

**Well-Meaning People**

Then, of course, there are the well-intentioned people who want to help but can sometimes do more harm than good. Let me give two examples of actions that have been hurtful in my own experience.

First is what I call *minimizing.* It goes something like this. When someone asks how I am doing, I tell him or her I have trouble sleeping and I often have trouble with short-term memory. A common response is, "Hey, we're all getting older and just the other day I got into the car to go somewhere and forgot where I was going." Though people want to identify with the person who is suffering, what they are actually doing is *minimizing* what the person is going through, as though it was something normal or age-related. In others words, it's no big deal.

Another hurtful response is what I call *comparing.* Sometimes when I tell somebody about a certain symptom I am experiencing, I often get this response: "I know a guy ..." and they proceed to tell me about somebody they know who had similar symptoms. And in some cases, they even go so far as to prescribe a treatment! Then, of course, there are those individuals who are experts on every subject. If these folks have a spiritual gift, it must be the gift of discouragement.

**The Devil's Tool**

The story is told that the devil decided to have a garage sale. Taking out all his finest tools of deception and death, he priced and placed each one on the driveway. They were each marked according to their value. There was hatred, envy and jealousy all marked for sale. There was deceit, lust, lying and pride with their appropriate price tags.

But, set over by itself, totally removed from the other instruments, was an unassuming plain-looking tool. It was quite worn. In fact, it was the most worn of all the tools, and yet it carried the highest price. A customer sauntered up and began browsing through the tools. He picked it up, looked it over, and casually asked the devil, "Say, what's the name of this tool?"

With a shrewd sneer, the devil boldly replied, "Ahh, my favorite tool. I know it well. That's the tool called discouragement."

"Is that high price negotiable?" the customer asked.

"No, absolutely not. That tool is more powerful than any other tool I have. When I use the tool of discouragement on a person's heart, I can pry open that person's heart and then use all of my other tools. It is the key tool—my most strategic tool—and therefore comes at a very high price."[1]

That little parable contains a lot of truth. Family and friends have the potential to help us or hurt us. They can lift us up or put us down.

Those who encourage us are special people in our lives. One special joy I've had has been the reintroduction of my brother-in-law into my life. My sister Jeanette married Ron when I was in high school and they moved to Oklahoma where Ron and his family were from. Now, thirty years later, I have wound up living in the same town as Ron and Jeanette. Ron and I like to drink coffee. He will call me on a regular basis and we meet at our hangout to just talk for an hour or so. He is always an encouragement.

**Pamala:** Richard and I were hurt deeply by a few close friends and family members as we entered into the early stages of this disease, simply because they could not understand it. Sometimes what we cannot understand makes us afraid, and with this fear comes things like denial, rejection, abandonment, neglect, guilt and blame. I don't think these people intentionally said or wanted to do the wrong things, but nevertheless, they did. We received critical advice from them when what we needed was a helping hand and loving heart. Fortunately for us, there was a whole group of friends and family who did take on the responsibility to lovingly support us even when we were more of a liability than an asset. *Thank you.*

There are times when being a friend takes courage. Our friends have been put to the test during these five years of Richard's illness. When Richard first started having symptoms those of us close to him were at a loss as to why he would behave in such an uncharacteristic way. I poured my heart out to great friends like Kay and Tricia, Tina, Eddie and Lance—all of them promising prayers, loyalty, compassion and commitment to us through whatever lay ahead. Friends like ours have remained great encouragers and have partnered hand in hand with us on this road of suffering in slow motion.

Perhaps you would like to be the kind of friend who encourages and is truly supportive of a family in the midst of their suffering, but you are unsure what to do or how you should go about it. Richard and I have put together a helpful "to do" and "not to do" list for those who truly want to help. God made our hearts to love; without love from family and friends life will be long and lonely here on earth.

Please take time to look over the suggestions below, choose

a few that you can implement in the life of a person or family in need. Someone desperately needs your love in action today.

1. When asking, "How are you?" refuse to accept a "fine" answer. Always follow up with another question. Probe, without prying, for the truth.

2. Work to keep in touch throughout the longevity of the illness. Don't quit. Too often the "out of sight, out of mind" rule applies. It takes work to be a true friend. "There are 'friends' who destroy each other, but a real friend sticks closer than a brother" (Prv 18:24, NLT). Job himself said, "A despairing man should have the devotion of his friends, even though he forsakes the fear of the Almighty" (6:14).

3. Send an Email or card (humorous as well as inspirational).

4. Telephone them. A short conversation is all that is needed.

5. Be the aggressor in the friendship. Just dealing with the stress of an illness takes so much energy that little is left to seek out the much-needed friendships at this time. Proverbs 17:17 states, "A friend loves at all times, and a brother is born for adversity."

6. Be thoughtful. Offer to pick up some groceries or a pizza, scrub a shower, rake the leaves, etc. Look for practical ways to help and then do them. Most people in need are not very comfortable asking for help.

7. Include their family in as many social activities as you can. Exclusion and isolation are common problems for the healthy members of the family.

8. Remember to check on the caregiver. Ask how *they* are doing and offer to take them out on occasion.

9. Be on their side. Do not criticize them or the decisions they must make. Unless you have personally been in their exact situation, you really don't know what you would do if you were in their shoes.

10. Listen more than you talk. Sometimes all that is needed is companionship. Take something you can do with your friend. Perhaps you can just sit and read to them, rent a movie, or listen to their favorite music.

11. Offer hope with love and compassion, not judgment or criticism.

12. Say something about the fact that they are suffering. Ignoring the obvious is awkward. Say, "I wish I knew the right thing to say, but I care and I am here if you need me."

13. Pray for them and their family. Pray for courage, energy, rest, peace and for their specific needs like financial resources, wisdom, understanding, coping with pain, etc. "Carry each other's burdens, and in this way you will fulfill the law of Christ" (Gal 6:2).

14. Try to exude joy in their presence; smiles are contagious!

15. Avoid telling them what you would do if you were in their shoes.

16. Don't feel compelled to share every "cure" you've heard of for their illness. It's insulting and implies that they haven't been doing their own "homework."

17. Be aware of the fact that illness is not just a matter of attitude. Beware of telling people that they just need to have more faith.

18. Respect their limitations. Unless you are the person's therapist, don't try and push them beyond their comfort level.

19. Remember special occasions, like birthdays. You can always brighten somebody's day by simply remembering little things.

20. **DWYSYWD**. That's short for "Do what you said you would do." If you tell the person you will call them tomorrow, call them tomorrow. They are counting on you to keep your word.

### For Group Discussion:
1. Share an anonymous example of a *well-meaning* person.
2. What one attribute of a family member or friend has helped you the most?
3. Pick two suggestions from our list of twenty: one that would help you most and one you could use to help another person. Why did you make your particular choices?

**Personal Application:**

1. Are you allowing resentment to grow in your heart due to disappointment with family or friends? If so, how do you plan to deal with it?

2. Do you have someone that has *a shared lump in the throat* in your behalf? If so, take a few minutes to thank God in prayer for them.

3. Is there somebody God is calling you to befriend?

**Just For the Caregiver**

How could we ever underestimate the value of family and friends? On occasion people disappoint us, but so very often God uses another person at just the right time to meet a need in our lives. This week, maybe you can treat yourself to a favorite pastime with a friend, and find new energy and a renewed zeal to care for your loved one.

## TEN

## Making the Hard Decisions

**Pamala:** I never intended to be the one in charge of things in our family. I truly have had the Peter Pan mind-set—"I'll never grow up, no, never grow up." It was just fine for Richard to be the grown-up and give direction while I led the troops in having fun, kicking it up, smelling the roses, dancing and playing as much as possible. Actually, it was a great balance. Richard was fanatically driven and focused, so my planning the fun was crucial for his survival. He in return challenged me to take life more seriously. Never did we imagine our life circumstances would require a role reversal. But that's the thing about crises—they are never planned. That being the case, most of us will not be prepared when a crisis comes. The element of surprise was not a good thing in our case, but it was reality.

### Accepting Reality

My reality? I had to do some changing because of Richard's terminal illness. I had to be in charge of everything, including him. Caring for someone who is dying is a huge assignment. That in itself takes courage, energy, wisdom, patience and a good sense of humor. But all caregivers have other things to do besides. We have jobs to go to, kids to raise or parents who are dependent on us, or all of the above. Birthday parties and weddings still need to be attended; our show must go on.

That's the really extra-hard part for me. I didn't feel like I *deserved* to laugh and play while Richard suffered. How could I plan life while his plan for the near future was death? I resisted for a while. I stayed in, and shut the doors of our home and my heart. Our home became a tomb. There was no fun, no music, no noise and certainly no dancing. I was checking out with Richard—that is, until we had another unplanned crisis.

### Another Crisis

Our oldest child, Apryl, had a crisis of her own. She went into premature labor with her second child in the beginning of her seventh month. The doctor tried to stop her labor, but within a couple of days our very little Jewel Katelynn decided it was time to arrive on the scene and save us all. I say save us because her birth did just that.

Because of some emotional, spiritual and medical problems, Apryl needed some time off. And I was not about to let anyone else take care of her new baby and her four-year-old daughter, Chelsea. That was my assignment. The girls would live with us while Apryl spent time putting her life back together. I would not call this perfect timing because Richard was dealing with major depression over his recent diagnosis; Aaron, our son, was just entering high school; and our middle child, Amy, was graduating from the University of Washington and moving back home.

Having Apryl's girls move into our home took some adjustment since we lived in a three-bedroom garden home. You know, the one you buy to downsize? Little did we know the challenges that *upsizing* would bring our way.

Chelsea slept in her own special little area in our bedroom, while at the foot of our bed a bassinet awaited Jewel's release from the hospital. She would be in the neo-natal unit of the hospital for two months. During those two months I would go to the hospital three to four times a day to hold and feed her. It was a necessity for the growth and development of a pre-mature baby.

Jewel was finally released the day after Thanksgiving, a day I will cherish always. The moment this little girl came into our home, the house that had been becoming a tomb for the living instantly changed—new life had been breathed into it! God gave Jewel to all of us as a reminder that life is precious and has a way of going on.

God had to force me to look into the future—Richard's and mine—in an eternal sense of the word. Jewel was part of us, something eternal the two of us had started when her mother, Apryl, was conceived. Each time I looked into Jewel's choco-late brown eyes, I saw Richard. I could not help but see that part of him would continue to live on in my lifetime, as well as long after I am gone.

Now as I observe each of our children and grandchildren, I see a glimpse of Richard. It has brought me joy and comfort. It has also given me courage and cause to live on. However, even after I snapped out of my tomblike attitude, I would still be faced with other challenges.

**Guilt**

If someone you love is suffering, there will be times you will feel guilty. Guilt when you see them suffering and you are helpless to ease it. Guilt over a fun evening with friends when you know your loved one is at home not having any fun. Guilt over planning for the future that will not include them. Guilt for feeling lonely and wishing or praying for this long suffering to be over, for God to take them. Guilt for not loving them the same way you once did. Guilt for hard decisions you must make on their behalf.

## Decisions

Making decisions for another person, especially for an adult, is a big responsibility. But there will probably be a time when you as a caregiver will be forced to make some decisions for your loved one. In our case I had to set limits on what Richard could and could not do. In the beginning it was small things, like cutting back on his hours at work. But as Richard's illness progressed, things got more complicated. When he got to the point where he could easily get involved in road rage, or spend an enormous amount of money and not even remember what he had purchased, I had to take away his keys and say, "No driving," and take away the checkbook and say, "No spending." Taking the keys and checkbook from Richard was the right thing to do for his safety and for our financial future, but it was humiliating for him and enormously difficult for me.

## Medication and Treatment

Other hard decisions I had to make were about medication and treatment. The meds that are prescribed for Richard are very expensive and not covered by insurance, because they are not proven to actually help his condition. We have had more trial-and-error in this area than I want to recall. Since

Richard's disease is relatively rare, we have been forced to try certain medications, then wait and see. This has been very frustrating for both of us. He would get to the point of saying, "No more." I would say, "Yes, one more." There are side effects to everything he is taking, but he is dying, so it matters less if it is hard on another part of his body.

We are seeking some quality of life while he still has life. I cannot emphasize this enough: As long as there is life, it is important to make it as good as possible. This will require you—the caregiver—to make many decisions about medications, limitations and the type of care that is needed. No one can assume the responsibility of making these decisions except the daily caregiver. The caregiver lives with the daily challenge of making life as good as possible—for everyone. The caregiver is the one who deals with the pain, sadness, frustration, hopelessness and, most of all, the reality of the disease on a daily basis. This is often with very little help or consideration from others. Other people may pop in and check on Richard. They may even call and take him out for an hour or two, but I am the one in charge of the other twenty-two hours of every day.

## Caregivers

The term "caregiver" refers to anyone who provides assistance to someone else who is in some degree incapacitated and needs help. It usually refers to unpaid individuals such as family members, friends and neighbors who provide care. I had not given the word much thought until I was in the role myself. I was forty-three when Richard began to be ill. For me it would be a progressive role, requiring me to provide more and more care as Richard's health deteriorated. For others it can immediately become a full-time role as the result of an accident or an occurrence at birth. Whatever the circumstances that cause you to take up the role of caregiver, it will demand time, energy, money, self-sacrifice and a strong support system from family and friends. And most of all, you will need God to enable you to fulfill the demands of being a caregiver.

Here are some interesting statistics about care giving:

- Fifty-two million American caregivers provide care to someone twenty or older, who is ill or disabled.[1]
- Nearly one out of every four households is involved in care giving to persons aged 50 or over.[2]
- Approximately 75 percent of those providing care to older family members and friends are female.[3]
- Some studies show a more equitable distribution of care giving between male and female. However, female caregivers spend fifty percent more time providing care than the male caregivers.[4]
- The person most likely to be providing care to an older person is a daughter.[5]
- A breakdown of who is taking on the roles of caregiver looks like this:

| Relationship to Older Person | Percent of All Caregivers |
|---|---|
| Wife | 13.4 percent |
| Husband | 10.0 |
| Daughter | 26.6 |
| Son | 14.7 |

Other female relative ................17.5

Other male relative......................8.6

Other female nonrelative ...........5.7

Other male nonrelative ..............1.8

- Number of hours of care provided: 73 hours per week (10.5 hours per day).[6]
- The duration of care giving can last from less than a year to over forty years. The majority of caregivers provide unpaid assistance for one to four years; twenty percent provide care for five years or longer.[7]
- Studies show that among caregivers an estimated forty-six to fifty-nine percent are clinically depressed.[8]
- Caregivers use prescriptions drugs for depression, anxiety and insomnia two to three times as often as the rest of the population.[9]
- The estimated value of informal care giving if services had to be replaced with paid services would cost an estimated $196 billion annually.[10]

As you well know, care giving is more than facts and statistics. But the one fact most often overlooked is the actual wear and tear on the caregiver. In his book *Adrenaline and Stress*, Dr. Archibald Hart writes: "Stress begins in the mind but ends in the body, and the heart is the central target of destruction for much of the harmful stress we experience."[11]

Dr. Hart goes on to list the effects of stress on various parts of the body:

- **Brain:** generalized panic and anxiety, migraine headaches.

- **Heart:** rapid heartbeat, skipped beats, raised blood pressure, thumping and mid-sternum mild pain, dizziness and light headedness from high blood pressure, palpitations.
- **Stomach and Intestines:** general gastric distress, feelings of nausea, acid stomach and heartburn, diarrhea (chronic and acute), some forms of colitis indigestion, constipation.
- **Muscles:** neck ache and shoulder pain, headaches, stiff neck, teeth grinding, jaw joint pain, high and low back pain, generalized pain in arms and legs.
- **Hands and Skin:** cold extremities, increased sweating, skin eruptions.
- **Lungs:** respiratory problems, some asthmas, hyperventilation, shortness of breath.
- **General:** feelings of "trembling," fear of impending doom, inability to sit long, squirming and fidgeting, foot tapping, pacing, feelings of fatigue and lack of energy or heaviness, heightened irritability and anger, racing thoughts, daydreaming, indecisiveness, sleep disruptions.[12]

The point is well established that in our decision making as caregivers, we must leave room and time to care for our own needs or soon we will be in the need of a caregiver too.

### Sideline Coaching From Well-Meaning Friends
Some well-meaning family and friends have criticized my decisions about medication and treatment for Richard. We have been sent bottles of minerals to drink, herbs to take, websites to visit, articles to read, diets to be on, faith healers to

seek, Bible verses to read and prayers of repentance to pray. I have tried most of the above, but when it came down to what really helped, I had to go with what worked best for us. That was a combination of trust in God, good doctors and the proper balance of medications. At times we have operated on a trial-and-error basis because the disease is still considered uncharted waters.

I want to help you let go of any guilt you may feel when it comes to your decisions about medication and treatment. Seek as much input from the experts as possible. Research each new drug. Try as many as you have energy and resources to try. But do what is best for both you and the person you are responsible for. It is not a comfortable place to be in, but it is yours. Take the responsibility with courage and confidence. God will give you both of these much-needed inner strengths if you ask Him. I trust in the verses that remind me that God will guide me, instruct me and give me peace (Is 50:10; Prv 4:6; Col 3:15).

## Living Arrangements

Another hard decision faces you when a change in living arrangements becomes necessary. This has proven to be the most difficult area of decision making for me. Of course, each illness and each individual case must be considered based on its own circumstances. No one answer will work for everyone. There is no set formula, so you just have to assess the need as it arises and make the best decision for all involved.

Richard's illness is a brain disease that requires regimented order in his surroundings and total control of his environment. Stimulus, noise and disruption of the order can cause him to become very agitated and aggressive in his behavior. It can also keep him from being able to sleep for many nights in a row. My son, Aaron, and I made great efforts to provide the needed atmosphere for Richard in our home, but in time it became impossible to carry it out.

In time, Richard reached the point in the illness that required him to live separately from us. He could no longer live in a normal family environment. At first I rejected this idea entirely. I had operated my life around Richard's disease for six years. I found it distressful to let him out of my sight and control. Taking care of him was my job, filling my life completely. After being together for twenty-seven years, I had no idea how to live without him here with me. I knew that moving him to a more suited environment was the right decision, the best one for him as well as for me and Aaron, but it was still frightening for me. We looked at all the options and made the best decision we could, given our circumstances. We decided to move Richard into Baptist Village, an assisted living facility that has graduated levels of care based on the person's need.

As it turns out, moving Richard has been the right decision. Richard's quality of life is better. Now, because he is less frustrated and less disrupted, our time together is better. I continue to take care of things for him and I see him every day if at all possible. On a good day, when he is more rested, I can take him to lunch or a movie, and our time is enjoyable. We are both at peace with this decision and fully understand how we got here.

I know that in time, as the disease progresses, full-time care will be needed. I will deal with that decision in the same way as with this most recent one. I will cry and resist as long as it's possible, but in the end, I will be brave and make the hard decision to place him in the best possible environment I can afford.

## Planning for Death

Another reality we have to face is the fact that sooner or later our loved one is going to die. Death always seems like a good thing to prepare for, even if there is no immediate concern that it is going to happen. But few of us actually plan ahead for death. In our case we have been told that death could come soon for Richard.

I would like to make the following suggestions for preparing for the death of someone we love so much. The Bible says we should rejoice at death and cry at birth. I must admit I have not been able to do that just yet, but I am preparing for what is ahead. As he indicated in a previous chapter, Richard has written his desires for his memorial service already, and we are in the process of completing many of the following steps:

- The first important step is to determine who's responsible for financial matters. It makes a difference because financial institutions will only recognize authorized individuals.

- Key roles to consider include the executor of an estate; a beneficiary of an insurance policy or retirement fund; the holder of a power of attorney; a trustee; a joint owner of a bank account; or a cosigner on a loan or safe deposit box. You can have as many copies of a death certificate as you want, but if your name and signature are not on the safe deposit box account, you're not getting into that box without a court order.

- Speaking of the death certificate, you will need lots of them, and you will need them quickly. Most companies will need to have one to close out an account; insurance companies will require one to process a claim. Call the coroner's office in the community where the person passed away. If they don't handle it there, they can tell you who does.

- If you're the executor of the person's estate, it's your job to pay any outstanding debts and disperse any remaining funds or property to the beneficiaries listed in the will.[13]

I admit that by nature I do not like taking charge and making hard decisions. But I have found that I can do it and I feel I am doing a good job given my circumstances. If you are a caregiver, ask God for new courage to do the things required for this "unsolicited position" you find yourself in now. I did, and I have discovered "I can do everything with the help of Christ who gives me the strength I need" (Phil 4:13, NLT).

**For Group Discussion:**
1. Are you feeling guilty over a decision you have made or need to make? If so, can you share it with the group?
2. If you are a caregiver, how much of your week is spent in tending to the needs of a loved one?
3. Have friends and family disagreed with some of your decisions? If so, how have you handled it?

## For Personal Application:

1. Are you putting off making some hard decisions? If so, list them and take them one at a time. Seek advice from trusted counsel and make your move.
2. Most caregivers flirt with exhaustion. Are you taking care of yourself? If someone offers to give you a break, do you refuse? It's OK to take some time for yourself.
3. Ask God today for His strength and courage to live life one day at a time.

## Just For the Caregiver

At the age of 43 Pamala was given the role of caregiver. Her life was drastically changed, just like many of you. Pamala did her homework to discover what giving care should look like, where to get help, and the kind of risks associated with care giving if one does not take of oneself. What are you doing to de-stress your daily life? Are you watching your diet? Do you have some form of exercise? How long since your last physical? Do not neglect your own needs, and do not go on a guilt trip for taking care of yourself. Practice letting go of expectations of others and do what you need to do. Only you can do this for yourself.

As a caregiver for a loved one, you are one special person. You may not feel that way, but it's true. Love that is self-sacrificing is the highest form of love. Anybody can be selfish; just look around. Your labor of love may go unnoticed by some, but God reserves a special love for those who tend to the needs of others (Mt 10:42).

## ELEVEN

## Prayer and Journaling: Seeking the Father's Heart

**Pamala:** The practice of prayer and journaling has been my greatest source of strength throughout this journey of suffering in slow motion. I will complete my eighteenth year of journaling at the end of this year. I had already been journaling, along with spending time in prayer, for eleven years prior to Richard's diagnosis. I know God wanted this discipline to be well formed in me so He could use it to strengthen my life when I would need it most.

Praying and the practice of journaling have kept me going when nothing else has. I admit, family and friends have their place to help and lift burdens along the way, but they are human and will at some point let you down. Even though they will try to be there for you as much as possible, they cannot be there for you 24/7. Only God can do that.

### Prayer Defined

I have been acquainted with "church" my entire life. My dad was a Baptist pastor and I learned early in life how to follow all the rules expected of a faithful churchgoer. One of those disciplines is prayer. However, eighteen years ago I had an experience that changed my perspective on prayer. I used to have the idea that prayer was spending about five or maybe even ten minutes giving God my list of things I wanted Him to do for me. I was wrong. Prayer is so much more than that. *Prayer is the awesome privilege we mortals have to talk with the most powerful Person in the universe—God, Himself—and to hear back from Him.* As I took hold of this truth, my approach to prayer radically changed.

Here's how the change took place. Though I could teach a Sunday school class, play the piano on Sundays for worship, direct the choir, plan a great church social, lead a Bible study and tell a person how to become a Christian, there was something missing. I knew everything about working hard for God. I figured I knew Him as well as anyone else—after all, I had spent my life doing stuff for Him. But my level of intimacy with God was challenged when a new Christian's pure faith was expressed openly one Sunday evening.

The woman's name is Cheryl. She stood up and gave a testimony that left me with many questions. She said nine months earlier in her prayer time God had revealed to her information about her husband's job situation. God had told her that there was going to be a change in his career. He told her the exact time and specifics about an increase in pay. Cheryl said that, in exactly nine months, what God had told her came true. She was excited and awed with the truth of God's word. As I sat there listening to her story I was perplexed. "Why her and not me, Lord? After all, she has known You only for a *year*—maybe two—and I have been working hard for You for many years. Why would You talk to her so intimately, like a friend, and not to me, too?" I needed to have this question answered. So the next morning, after getting the kids off to school, I got my Bible and got on my knees to pray.

I must say that this prayer was different than any of my previous prayers. I had no list to give God that day. I only had one question that I wanted answered. I did not approach Him in reverent formality. I just opened up my Bible and said very directly, "God, I want all of You that is mine to have. I have done everything I thought You wanted me to do. Now I just want You. I want Your presence; I want to have a real conversation with You. I have no idea if You actually communicate with us now like you did in the Bible, but if You do, I want to know how to do it. I want to know if You tell us things like Cheryl said, things about the future that only You know about. Do You still do that?" Then I lay my head down on the Bible, asking God to please answer me.

I waited there listening, really expecting an answer. As I waited I heard within my spirit a quiet voice tell me to begin reading my Bible. I opened it and started reading where I had left off a few days earlier. It was Isaiah 42:8: "I am the Lord; that is my name! I will not give my glory to another or my praise to idols. See, the former things have taken place, and new things I declare; before they spring into being I announce them to you." First of all, He wanted me to know that it was Him talking to me. The text began, "I am the Lord!" And then He answered my question: *Yes, He does declare things before they happen!* That day I knew God spoke directly to me. I came to Him in faith, expecting Him to answer, and He did.

The great news is that God desires to communicate with everyone. We do not always need to know about the future, but at times we do. These types of answers to prayer build our faith and cause us to pray more expectantly. Many times we need to know what is up ahead so our hearts and our lives will be prepared. Jesus told His disciples on a regular basis that He was going to die and three days later He would come back to life again (Mk 10:33-34). He tried to prepare them and give them hope in the midst of what would seem like hopeless circumstances.

We can come to God with questions about anything. The answers do not always come quickly. Sometimes we must keep praying in faith and with persistence. God's answer to your request could be a "Yes," giving you reason to dance. Or it could be "No, I have a *better* plan, a *different* plan." But in time there will always be an answer.

## Praying for Specific Needs

Carol recently moved to Oklahoma from California. She was feeling lonely and sad, and so she asked God to give her at least one person who could understand what she had left behind and her life's work for the past twenty years. The very next morning at a coffee shop Carol and her husband, Steve, mentioned to a stranger that they had just moved here from California. The stranger pointed to a woman across the room and told them that woman was also from California. You guessed it—that woman was me! Steve and Carol approached me and it didn't take long to discover we had much more in common than moving from California to Oklahoma. She had worked for a Christian music publisher and we shared similar ministry experiences. We also discovered we were raised in the same Baptist denomination and our families had known each other for many years. Carol had a specific need; she expressed that need to God, knowing that He could help her. She left it up to Him to meet that need in the way He chose. (I forgot to tell you that my 9:30 A.M. class had been cancelled that day and I was killing some time.)

I am convinced there are some things that will never happen unless we ask. There are treasures that will not be found unless we seek, and there are doors that will remain closed unless we knock. Though we are participants in the process, we do not direct it. God hears and will answer our cry for help. He knew where I was going to be that day in the restaurant before I did. He directed Carol's steps to me. We have already been blessed by this new friendship. There is nothing too big or too small to ask of God.

### Praying to Accomplish God's Will

The late Dr. John Peters founded World Neighbors, a phenomenal mission organization, in the 1950s after hearing God's specific call. He was instructed by God to help less fortunate people by offering a "hand up instead of a handout."

Loren Cunningham began Youth With A Mission (YWAM) through an outright supernatural encounter with God. Loren's vision has materialized into a worldwide ministry that has sent out more than 15,000 workers each year helping people in more than two hundred different countries. My daughter Amy, at the age of 14, asked God to provide her the money she needed for a summer mission trip. He gave her exactly what she needed through a summer babysitting job.

God calls to the young and the older, more mature believer alike. They all hear a call from God to reach out to others in His name. He is available to everyone equally. "This is the confidence we have in approaching God: that if we ask anything according to his will, he hears us. And if we know that he hears us—whatever we ask—we know that we have what we asked of him" (1 Jn 5:14-15).

Your question may be, "How can I know if I am asking according to God's will?" Good question. In his book, *Is That Really You, God?*, Loren Cunningham makes these suggestions when seeking to know God's will:

- Submit to His lordship; silence your own thoughts, desires and the opinions of others.
- Allow God to speak to you in the way He chooses. Do not try to dictate to Him concerning methods.
- The methods He commonly uses are: the Bible, the inner voice, circumstances, and peace while praying.
- Obey the last thing He told you before moving forward.
- Do not talk about what God said to you until He gives you permission to do so. This is to avoid pride, pre-sumption, and confusion among others who are not ready to receive what God has said to you.
- Be aware of counterfeits like Ouija boards, séances, for-tune-telling and astrology. The guidance from God will lead you closer to Jesus and true freedom. Other forms will lead you away from God and into bondage.

Remember, relationship is the most important reason for hearing the voice of God. True guidance is getting closer to the guide.[1]

## The Prayer of Intercession

The term *intercession* literally means "to come between." To intercede in prayer is to stand between God and another per-son. This type of prayer is actually the fruit of a desire God places within the heart of a person to pray fervently for another. The intercessor may feel a special "burden" to pray for another and, through prayer, "stands in the gap" between God and the other person. Intercession takes the person's need and places it with our powerful God to do something about it. The person being prayed for may never know the intercessor is praying for them.

I have been given this type of prayer burden only twice in my life. There are times when I have felt such a heaviness in my heart to pray for an individual that it would wake me up in the middle of the night. It would keep me praying until I felt some reassurance that all was well.

This type of praying takes a great amount of discipline and faith. At times I have felt inconvenienced and grown weary at the lack of change or response I've seen in the people I have prayed for. But we must be willing to take our hands off and allow God to work as He chooses in their lives. It is an awesome thing to be trusted to pray for someone in this manner. Listen to these precise instructions: "I urge, then, first of all, that requests, prayers, intercession and thanksgiving be made for everyone—for kings and all those in authority, that we may live peaceful and quiet lives in all godliness and holiness. This is good, and pleases God our Savior, who wants all men to be saved and to come to a knowledge of the truth" (1 Tm 2:1-4).

## Prayers for Healing

**Richard:** Does God heal today? Or, an even more relevant question is, will God heal me? It's easy to theorize about suffering when you're not doing any. But when it comes knocking at your door, it's a whole new ball game. As Ron Dunn has said, "Pain can make us desperate."[2]

Let me assure you that I believe in divine healing. I believe that all healing is divine, whether it comes at the hand of a skilled surgeon, prescription drugs or an intervention of God without the assistance of another person or substance. While there are no guarantees, it is always right to ask God to heal us.

Should we pray for others when they are sick? Definitely. For ourselves when we are sick? Absolutely. First, "Let your requests be made known," the Bible tells us (Phil 4:6, KVJ). Ask. Be specific. We are admonished, "Do not be anxious about anything, but in everything, by prayer and petition, with thanksgiving, present your requests to God" (Phil 4:6). Prayer is a mystery and God invites us to be a part of it.

Second, we must be willing to submit to the Father's will. Here, again, Jesus leads the way. "Yet not as I will, but as you will" (Mt 26:39). Wanting what God wants more than what I want has always been the toughest part of following Jesus. But it is the very essence of being a Christ-follower. It's what following Jesus is all about. I know the personal angst of wondering what God is doing in my life and why He doesn't make everything better. He will. It's only a matter of time.

Third, we need to explore the depths of God's grace. Grace is more than a prayer at mealtime. Grace is one of those often-used words that is rarely understood. At its core it means lovingkindness, or favor. To experience God's grace means to come to the knowledge that you are the object of God's favor. He loves you—and He even *likes* you! Grace is like a life preserver. Imagine you are on a boat and you fall overboard. You would prefer to get back into the boat, right? But the next best thing is to have a life preserver to cling to until you can be rescued. Grace is God's provision for our overboard experiences,

His pledge to us that His grace will be sufficient, adequate, enough.

## Prayers of Gratefulness

**Pamala:** Prayer is talking to God about what is in your heart. Hopefully you can express love and adoration for God as well as your need for His care. I especially enjoy the times my children tell me they love me and do not ask for one thing. I love when they call just to say "hi" and say they miss me. Likewise, I am certain God enjoys this kind of love from His kids.

Sometimes prayer should just be about gratefulness. Take time to say "thank you" to God. The Bible says in 1 Chronicles 16:8-12: "Give thanks to the Lord, call on his name; make known among the nations what he has done. Sing to him, sing praise to him; tell of all his wonderful acts ... let the hearts of those who seek the Lord rejoice.... Seek his face always.... Remember the wonders he has done, his miracles." Take time to simply say, "I love you, God. Thank You for all of my blessings."

## Honest Prayers

There will be times when you are confused by what God seems to be doing—or not doing. Tell Him what's on your mind. You can say anything to Him; He is big enough to take it. So go ahead—dish it out. Certainly I have had moments of anger, questioning why God has allowed suffering and tragedy to come to our family. I do not have the complete answer yet, but I do know He wants me to know a supernatural peace, comfort, strength and joy that is always available, even during lengthy times of suffering.

In difficult times it is OK to ask God, "Why?" King David did. "How long must I wrestle with my thoughts and every day have sorrow in my heart?" (Ps 13:2). Jesus, Himself, asked the Father a similar question: "My God, my God, why have you forsaken me?" (Mt 27:46). God never seems offended by anyone asking Him "Why?" He just wants us to talk to Him about what is in our heart. Many times, I can see that my children are upset even before they tell me. I usually already know what the problem is, but I still love it when they trust me enough to come and share their troubles, their questions and their needs. I love it when we can talk about these things together. God also wants us to come to Him when we are angry or confused. He has brought me comfort, even if my circumstances did not change. There are times we must trust the fact that He is God and we are not. His ways are higher than ours and we must rest in the knowledge that He is going to work all things for our good in the end.

"Ask and it will be given to you; seek and you will find; knock and the door will be opened to you. For everyone who asks receives; he who seeks finds; and to him who knocks, the door will be opened" (Mt 7:7-8). Notice that this verse urges us to be proactive. Prayer is not passive; it's aggressive. The verse implies consistency. We are instructed to keep on asking, seeking and knocking until the answer comes. I know my own children can be relentless when they want me to do something for them. When Amy was young she would tug at my arm until I would stop and listen to her. How wonderful that God is never too busy to listen to us. He loves it when we continue to come and spend time with Him.

In times of aloneness, suffering and sadness, God wants to

comfort you and me. To think that He is listening and available 24/7 is beyond my human understanding. I do not know how prayer works; I just know that it does. You do not need magic words, a special formula or access code; simply call out His name. He is listening.

## Journaling a Record

A part of my prayer experience is time spent writing in a journal. I don't start with "Dear Diary," but it is very much like a diary. Journaling is a record of your thoughts, prayer requests, an account of your daily activities, as well as a record of what God is doing in your life. Without some form of records, valuable proof is missing. Records are indispensable. Birth certificates, marriage licenses, drivers' licenses, death certificates and court proceedings are all valuable records. A journal is a similar document. I journal for several reasons:

- I want to look back and be reminded of all the wonders in my life.
- It reminds me that I am making progress.
- I get to see answers to my prayers and how long I prayed for someone or something.
- It is also great therapy. I can vent pretty well on paper.
- I am encouraged when I read how God lifted me up on a sad day by bringing a wonderful surprise into my life. I seem to have a bad memory on my own. My journal serves as a reminder of God's goodness.
- It serves as a record of those moments in life you want to always remember.

Journaling can be done anytime. All you need is paper and a pen. Or perhaps you prefer to use your computer, like Richard. He started using his computer to journal soon after he was diagnosed with his illness. Because of his journal entries, we have a large part of this book to share with you. I have all of my journals for the past eighteen years except one that I left on an airplane last Christmas. I tried for weeks and weeks to find it. I felt like I had lost a year of memories.

My first journal was a book of blank pages. I could write in it anytime I felt like it. Then I started being more accountable to myself, using a journal with dates in it. I could see how many days I had kept up with my journal and how many days I had skipped. I now have such a love for my journaling time that I rarely, if ever, miss a day in an entire year. I now prefer to use a journal that has a short inspirational message and room provided for me to respond to the message. I have found, time after time, that I needed exactly what was written on that day. It has sometimes been as if it was written just for me. I know God has used this discipline to guide me, show me His love, answer questions, correct wrong thinking and convict me of sin in my life. I strongly encourage you to get a journal that comes with some type of daily message or challenge. It can help you begin this discipline by giving you something to reflect on and write about.

But the most important thing about journaling is to do it. Journaling will become your record of growth, strength and courage through the good and bad times of your life. There are times I am proud as I read of my steps forward, and other times I am embarrassed at the life I see on the pages of my journal. My life can look a lot like a ship on a raging sea: lost, scared and coming apart at the seams. It's all there for me to reflect on. I am thankful I have both the good and the bad written down. I have found that it is during the raging storms of my life that I have learned the most, changed the most and become a stronger, better person.

**For Group Discussion:**

1. Is listening a regular part of your prayer time?
2. Can you share specific answers to specific prayers with the group? Tell us about them.
3. Loren Cunningham makes several points about how to discern God's will for our lives. Which one (or two) is the most meaningful to you?

**For Personal Application:**

1. Have you been able to pray the prayer of gratefulness, even in your time of sorrow? Reflect on 1 Chronicles 16:8-12 and write your thoughts in your journal.
2. Has God spoken to you about taking a specific action? Have you obeyed Him? Why or why not?
3. What practical steps can you take this week to seek the Father's heart? Write down your thoughts and reflect on them every day this week.

**Just For the Caregiver**

Much of what is written in this book would be inaccessible if it were not for Richard's journals. Pamala has kept a daily prayer journal now for eighteen years. Nothing can take the place of prayer and seeking the heart of God. For the caregiver, every new day brings the same heavy load as the day before—and maybe even a new weight.

Today could be the first day of a new discipline of writing a few lines in a journal. It can be in the form of a prayer; it can chronicle your thoughts or emotions; it can simply be a list of the anxieties you are facing. Don't set the bar at seven days a week; just begin with a goal of three or four days a week and go from there. But do it.

## TWELVE

## The Long View: Keeping Your Eyes on the Horizon

**Richard:** I was standing around in church before it began, talking with a couple who were manning their posts next to a ministry booth. (You know the kind, looking for new recruits.) At first we talked about general things, but then the woman asked what had brought me to the town where I am now living. I gave her the thirty-second version. No one had ever asked me before. She responded to my explanation with another question: "Now that you have been diagnosed with a terminal illness, how has it affected your view of the future?"

Several things raced through my mind at the same time. First, I thought, "You don't even know me, lady!" Then I thought, "That is a pretty good question. I wonder why nobody else has asked me that before." I attempted an honest answer. I told her it had been a mixture of grief and anticipation for what God has in store for me in the future. I told her it was time for me to practice what I had preached. She seemed satisfied with my answer.

### Is There Really a Heaven?

In the Christian tradition, the terms "heaven" and "hell" are powerful expressions of the immense privilege of fellowship with God and the awfulness of eternal separation from His presence. I think it is important for us to reflect on some of the key scriptural texts that shed light on this important subject. Why? Because what I think or say about the subject doesn't really matter. I wouldn't take another person's word on such an all-important subject. I want to hear it from God Himself.

Solomon said, "He [God] has planted eternity in the human heart" (Eccl 3:11, NLT). Perhaps that is part of what it means to be made in the image of God. There is a part of us that longs for wrongs to be made right, for righteousness to prevail over evil and for meaning to conquer meaninglessness. In His infinite wisdom God has a plan for the ages and a purpose for each of our lives.

### Some General Observations

The Bible speaks of heaven as God's home (Dt 26:15; Ps 2:4) and as the abode of angels (Mk 12:25; Lk 2:15). However, God is not restricted to heaven, for His presence fills creation (Ps 139:7-12). Here are some other facts Scripture tells us about heaven:

- Heaven is the place of perfection, where there is complete harmony and order (Lk 12:33; 1 Pt 1:4; Rv 21:10–22:5), and the realm in which God's will is perfectly done (Mt 6:10).
- The resurrected Christ returned to heaven (Acts 1:11) and from it He will come again for judgment (2 Thes 1:6-10) and to renew the world (2 Pt 3:13; Rv 21:1).
- In its final form as "the new heaven and new earth," heaven will be populated by believers having resurrected bodies (2 Cor 5:1-8). "God himself will be with them. He will remove all of their sorrows, and there will be no more death or sorrow or crying or pain. For the old world and its evils are gone forever" (Rv 21:3,4, NLT).

## An Up Close and Personal Observation

**Pamala:** For some people heaven can seem "way out there," but for me, it has become "up close and personal." Three years ago I had a horrendous accident in which I broke five vertebrae and crushed six discs in my neck and lower back. Several specialists told me I was "Humpty Dumpty" and could not be put back together again. This is not what I wanted to hear, nor did I believe God wanted me in a wheelchair for the rest of my life. After a long search, I discovered a group of doctors in Northern California who specialized in spinal reconstruction. They took my case believing I was an excellent candidate for the surgery and they expected it to be very successful. They informed me it would be about a ten-hour surgery and a long recovery.

I was convinced God was directing me to proceed with the surgery even though it would take a lot of effort to set things up for Richard's care in my absence. Our daughter Amy consented to move into our house to look after her dad and brother while I was in California undergoing the surgery. Everything fell into place and I was on my way to California for the operation.

The morning of the surgery I felt good, confident. The surgeons came in and assured me they were certain all would go well and had scheduled nine holes of golf for later that day. But they never made that tee time.

About half way into the surgery I began to experience loss of blood pressure. My back was opened up and nerves exposed—not a good time for things to become complicated. The anesthesiologist began the procedure to bring my pressure up, but with no success. Finally they decided that I must be losing blood from a major organ. This meant they needed to call in a vascular surgeon to go in and "look around." While they were bringing me out of the deep sleep and attempting to *flip me over* for the vascular surgeon, I could hear them talking frantically, almost yelling. The doctors were saying things like, "We're losing her!" "Hurry, she's not responding!" I remember it perfectly. Hysterical thoughts were racing through my mind. I cried to myself, "I'm dying, oh God, who will take care of the girls?" referring to my granddaughters Chelsea and Jewel. God said to me, "Pamala, I have them in my hands now and always." With that I was overcome by a great peace and, in fact, I died.

I know I died. I had never read an account of anyone dying. This experience was not a dream—it was real; it was true; it happened to me. I was walking through a very dark tunnel toward an intense light. The light was like a million sparklers—you know, the ones the kids play with on the Fourth of July. I was walking through this dark tunnel into the bright sparkling light. I remember feeling a peace that is beyond any known to me before. There are not sufficient words to describe this peace. I could see I was headed to the doorway of heaven. It was beautiful. I was not afraid; I was filled with joy! Just as I got close to the light I felt a hand on my left shoulder and then I heard a voice say, "Pamala, it is not time for you to go, my child." I knew it was the voice of Jesus. He took His hand and gently turned me around, and with that, I awoke in the recovery room. I had no idea that several days had passed. At the time I could not speak so I motioned for my friend Tricia to give me something to write with. I was very weak but managed to write, "I died." She looked at me puzzled and said, "You died? You will have to tell me all about that later!"

When I was able to speak I did tell her and other family members about the entire experience. It was about day nine when the doctor came into my room and said, "Pamala, I need to tell you about something that happened during your surgery." I looked at him, smiled and said, "I died, didn't I?" He looked a little upset and asked me who had told me. I got the opportunity to describe the entire experience to him in detail. I know he was perplexed by what I had to say, because there was no way for me to know what had gone on during surgery without someone telling me. I had indeed died and recalled the entire incident; no one could explain otherwise.

Why? Why did I die, remember it perfectly and come back to this life? Perhaps to tell this story to you or help others at the hospital have a deeper faith in God, or give validity of the afterlife to skeptics. I cannot say for certain, but I do believe God gave this particular experience to me to help Richard and our family as we face Richard's ominous future. Richard loves to listen to the story when he becomes anxious. I have told it repeatedly to our kids and grandkids when they seem fearful about death. From what I got a glimpse of, there is absolutely nothing to fear if heaven is where you are headed. Heaven is a place of magnificent beauty, euphoric peace, indescribable joy, and is bursting with happiness. I know; I experienced it up close and personal. The Bible tells us we should actually cry at the birth of a baby and rejoice over the death of a Christian (Eccl 7:1). I do not think our family is quite ready to rejoice, but I can say we are not frightened of death anymore.

All of us are terminal, when you think about it. Some are told when they can expect to die. Others may get surprised by it, like I did. But death is inevitable. Knowing God the Creator personally through His Son Jesus Christ will assure you and me a place in heaven forever. Heaven is real, I can assure you! Do you have that hope?

## The Hope of Heaven

**Richard:** Though it is "out there" in the future, contemplating heaven has profound implications for living here and now. Consider the following:

- It is a reminder to believers, as I noted, that we are "aliens and strangers in the world" (1 Pt 2:11). We are to cultivate a certain sense of spiritual detachment from this present world. As one gospel song reminds us, "This world is not my home; I'm just a passin' through."
- It is a reminder that "our citizenship is in heaven" (Phil 3:20). As believers we hold a *dual* citizenship. We are citizens of the country in which we were born and we are also citizens of God's family forever.
- It gives us hope "that our present sufferings are not worth comparing with the glory that will be revealed in us" (Rom 8:18). To those who suffer, it gives us a focal point for the future. It does not deny that our suffering is real, but in comparison, the glory to come will remove all tears and sorrow.
- It helps us to resist the temptation to lose heart. "Therefore we do not lose heart" (2 Cor 4:16). Losing heart is one of our greatest struggles. When we are phys-

ically weak it is so easy to lose heart. When we have suffered a tragic loss it is difficult to *take* heart.

- "Our *light* and *momentary* troubles are achieving for us an eternal glory that far outweighs them all" (2 Cor 4:17, emphasis added). Again, that is not to minimize our suffering, but to show the glorious contrast of what God has in store for those who love Him.

- Heaven will be eternal in duration. "Now we know that if the earthly tent we live in is destroyed, we have a building from God, an eternal house in heaven, not built by human hands" (2 Cor 5:1).

- God has given us a deposit to assure us of the reality of what is to come. "Now it is God who has made us for this very purpose and has given us the Spirit as a deposit, guaranteeing what is to come" (2 Cor 5:5).

When will I go to heaven? When will you go to heaven? I don't know the answer to that question, but I do know that we can trust God with our eternal destiny. He spared no expense to redeem us to Himself. He locked down His promise by the death and resurrection of His own Son and by the deposit of the Holy Spirit within us. God intends to gather us to Himself. It's only a matter of time.

**Earthlings**

So what keeps us from letting heaven fill our thoughts? What causes us to lose sight of what God has in store for us in the future? Let's see if we can answer that question. I think there is a triple threat to a heaven-filled thought life. The very fact that we are "here" and heaven is "there" is a good place to begin. We are earthlings, or as Peter said, *strangers* and *aliens*. All we know from firsthand experience is life here on this earth. And frankly, living here can cause us to lose perspective very easily.

In aeronautical terms losing sight of the horizon is referred to as spatial disorientation, and it can be a killer. According to flight training manuals, the eyes can help determine the speed and direction of flight by comparing the position of the aircraft relative to some fixed point of reference. Eighty percent of our orientation information comes from the visual system.

The most well-known, recent spatial disorientation disaster was the plane crash of John F. Kennedy Jr. The report published by the National Transportation Safety Board (NTSB) blamed the crash on "spatial disorientation, confusion in the brain that results from a loss of balance in the inner ear." Contributing to Kennedy's disorientation, the report said, were the night sky, a lack of visible horizon over the open water and a haze that blanketed Kennedy's flight path. When spatial disorientation occurs, a pilot who doesn't have any visual references may have difficulty determining whether the plane is climbing, descending or in a turn. While Kennedy's instincts told him he was flying parallel with the ground, his airplane's rate of descent eventually exceeded 4,700 feet per minute, and the airplane struck the water in a nose-down attitude. Unfortunately Kennedy had not yet completed his instrument rating.

When illness or tragedy strikes, disorientation is likely to follow. We lose our balance and our sense of equilibrium. The props are knocked out from under us. In a very real sense we suffer from our own version of spatial disorientation. Up seems like down and our lives are spinning out of control. Sometimes we can locate that point of reference on the horizon. At other times we have to trust God and fly by "instrumentation." Our tendency is to use our feelings as our guide. But oftentimes feelings are misleading.

## Materialism

In His Sermon on the Mount Jesus gave us a second clue about why our thoughts are often filled with things other than heaven. "Don't store up treasures here on earth, where they can be eaten by moths and get rusty, and where thieves break in and steal. Store your treasures in *heaven*, where they will never become moth-eaten or rusty and where they will be safe from thieves. Wherever your treasure is, there your heart and *thoughts* will also be" (Mt 6:19-21, NLT, emphasis added). This truth has been made so very sobering in light of the attack on America on September 11, 2001, and the collapse of the likes of Enron and WorldCom. I don't think Jesus is opposed to our investing in the stock market, but He is cautioning us about what we consider our "treasure." If all of our treasures are in stocks and bonds, we are headed for trouble.

## Worry

A third clue comes from Jesus' same sermon. "So don't *worry* about having enough food or drink or clothing. Why be like the pagans who are so deeply concerned about these things? Your heavenly Father already knows all your needs, and he will give you all you need from day to day if you live for him and make the Kingdom of God your primary concern. So don't *worry* about tomorrow, for tomorrow will bring its own *worries*.

Today's trouble is enough for today" (Mt 6:31-34, NLT, emphasis added).

## Finding a Solution

One conclusion we can draw from the teachings of Jesus is that filling our thoughts with heaven requires some "intentionality" on our part, right? Just as water seeks the lowest level, so our thoughts settle where we let them. Paul put it this way: "And now, dear brothers and sisters, let me say one more thing as I close this letter. Fix your thoughts on what is true and honorable and right. Think about things that are pure and lovely and admirable. Think about things that are excellent and worthy of praise. Keep putting into practice all you learned from me and heard from me and saw me doing, and the God of peace will be with you" (Phil 4:8-9, NLT).

Americans live in such a pressure-cooker lifestyle that when we get home from the office or the factory, we shift our minds into neutral. That usually means television or surfing the Internet. We allow our culture to take over our minds. We are mesmerized by the programming, not to mention the commercials. I'm not advocating that we abandon every form of entertainment, but I do believe we must take charge of our viewing minds. We need to be more discriminating in what we watch. We need to ask if it contributes to the categories of being true, honorable, right, excellent or worthy of praise?

To give me needed perspective, I have discovered that sitting and listening to my favorite Christian artist or reading large sections of Scripture out loud from several translations is of great value to me. In addition there are a host of Christian devotional guides on the market. And may I suggest the

Christian classics? Not those written in the past decade, but those written over the past century.

A second hindrance we identified was materialism. Materialism is simply wanting more than I have. That "new car" smell drives me nuts. Know what I mean? Jesus knew that getting overly concerned about our "stuff" would distract us and keep us from seeking the true treasures.

Perhaps a "treasure" inventory would be in order. Don't just look at stocks and bonds and other financial wealth in your portfolio, but also inventory those things that are intangible, those treasures like our pride, what other people think about public image, and so forth. For this inventory to be a success we must be ruthlessly honest. Only then will we be able to discern where our true treasures are and what captures the majority of our thoughts.

A third threat to having heaven-filled thoughts is anxiety. While there are various types of anxiety and different levels, I dare say that we all wrestle with anxiety and anxious feelings. Five times in His Sermon on the Mount Jesus referred to worry. Jesus didn't stop with just scolding His disciples, He admonished them to see how much the Father cares for all of His creation. He assured them that human life is more valuable to God than the plant and animal kingdoms. If God takes care of them, we should rest assured that He knows our needs and can take care of us.

Of course, some degree of fear and anxiety is perfectly normal. In the face of danger it prepares the body for the so-called "fight-flight" response. Specialists tell us that some people are genetically predisposed to anxiety. Other reasons like psychological trauma, stressful life events (e.g., the death of a loved one, divorce and the purchase of a mortgage!) can bring the all too familiar "butterflies in the stomach."

Of all the prescriptions and techniques I have seen, the one I liked best recommended "to put the anxiety out of one's mind by focusing thoughts on something else." Huh? That seems to be what Paul had in mind when he said, "Don't worry about anything; instead, pray about everything. Tell God what you need, and thank him for all he has done. If you do this, you will experience God's peace, which is far more wonderful than the human mind can understand. His peace will guard your hearts and minds as you live in Christ Jesus" (Phil 4:6-7, NLT). This text contains both a command and a promise. We are told not to worry, but rather, we are to pray about everything. If you're like me, when I am in a state of anxiety, prayer is often the last thing on my mind—and that is Paul's point here.

### The Promise of God's Peace

God's response to our cries should come as no surprise. "If you do this, you *will* experience God's peace" (Phil 4:7, NLT, emphasis added). Anxiety, as much as anything, will distract us and keep our thoughts from being filled with heaven.

Let's end where we began. What does it mean to have our thoughts filled with heaven? What does it mean to keep our eyes on the horizon? Does it mean to dwell on halos and harps? Hardly. At least in part, it means to consciously fix our thoughts on things that are eternal, things that are true and things that are honorable. As the writer of Hebrews exhorts us, it means to "fix our eyes on Jesus, the author and perfecter of our faith, who for the joy set before him endured the cross, scorning its shame, and sat down at the right hand of the throne of God" (12:2). The word "fix" (*aphorao*) means "to consider attentively."[1]

In the Old Testament this notion of fixed attention upon God and His Word was referred to as meditation. Listen to the words of the psalmist:

- "I meditate on your precepts and consider your ways. I delight in your decrees; I will not neglect your word" (Ps 119:15-16).
- "I lift up my hands to your commands, which I love, and I meditate on your decrees" (Ps 119:48).
- "I will meditate on all your works and consider all your mighty deeds" (Ps 77:12).
- "Oh, how I love your law! I meditate on it all day long. Your commands make me wiser than my enemies, for they are ever with me" (Ps 119:97-98).

You may feel clumsy at your first attempts at meditation, but all you have to lose is your anxiety! Peter (a rather clumsy guy himself) said, "Cast all your anxiety on him because he cares for you" (1 Pt 5:7). You may choose to play music softly in the background while you read through some of your favorite biblical texts, and rather than a "laundry list" approach to prayer, ask God to speak to you through His Word about your specific needs. Sit before Him in a period of silence. Sing a song of praise and worship to Him. Nothing can take the place of being attentive before God. Nothing.

To have our thoughts filled with heaven also means to be discerning and to learn to value things as God values them.

Our culture has switched the price tags of nearly everything, causing us to live in an upside-down world. Jesus told this story, "The kingdom of heaven is like treasure hidden in a field. When a man found it, he hid it again, and then in his joy went and sold all he had and bought that field" (Mt 13:44). Only as we find the true treasure will our lives be filled with satisfaction.

## For Group Discussion:

1. What aspect of heaven or eternal life gives you the most courage to keep pressing ahead?
2. What steps can you take (or have you taken) to help you focus on what God has in store for you in the future?
3. Share with the group how prayer has helped you with anxiety.

## For Personal Application:

1. Take a sheet of paper or a 3x5 card and write the words "My Fears" at the top. Take your time and list your fears. Next use your Fear Card as your Prayer Card for the coming week.
2. Read aloud to yourself the four Psalms (119:15, 16; 119:48; 77:12; 119:97, 98) that speak of the need to focus our minds on God's promises. Underline the words or thoughts that speak to you the most.
3. Write out a prayer to God requesting His peace.

## Just For the Caregiver

To some people, heaven is just a pipe dream or wishful thinking. To others of us it is a promise; a place that Jesus has gone to prepare for those who love Him. Just as sure as He came the first time, He said He would come again and take us home to be with Him (Jn 14:1-6).

God has room for you in His house. He has extended an invitation to you to join Him. "To all who received him [Jesus Christ], to those who believed in his name, he gave the right to become children of God" (Jn 1:12).

You can reserve a room in God's eternal dwelling place by praying a simple, heartfelt prayer such as this:

*Dear Lord Jesus, I confess to you my sin and shortcomings and my need for a Savior. I believe that You are God's only Son and only Savior for the world. I believe that You are the promised Messiah; that You came and offered your life as a sacrifice for my sin, and rose again on the third day. I receive You into my life today. Fill me with the hope that one day I will live in heaven with You forever, Amen.*

# In Summary

**Richard:** In the end it comes down to three things: faith, family and friends. My faith in God's sovereign plan for my life has helped me to stay the course, even when I can't see my way. But that's what trust is all about. My faith provides the hope that transcends all of my trials and fosters my belief that the best is yet to come. Paul wrote, "Therefore we do not lose heart. Though outwardly we are wasting away, yet inwardly we are being renewed day by day. For our light and momentary troubles are achieving for us an eternal glory *that far outweighs them all*" (2 Cor 4:16-17, emphasis added). God will more than make up for our trials here.

Nothing takes the place of family. Those individuals who love us unconditionally are God's gift to each of us. I am grateful to my own family for loving me as they do.

Pamala has been the ideal example of "in sickness and in health." Words could never describe her combination of courage and fortitude as well as her tenderness and gentle spirit. When I can no longer speak, Pamala, remember, you have been God's gift to my life.

My children and grandchildren have brought me joy beyond description. We have walked the road of life together. It has not always been easy, but we've always been together. We have refused to let people or things separate us. My heart will always treasure the memories of family vacations, holidays and driver's licenses. Your lives will go on. Stay in step with God and each other.

My friends have been a bonus in life. "If one falls down, his friend can help him up. But pity the man who falls and has no one to help him up" (Eccl 4:10)! I have done my share of falling down, but God has seen to it that there always has been a friend nearby. To my special friends (and you know who you are), I say "thank you" for your support when I stumbled, for your words of rebuke when I needed them, and for your steadfast love.

**Pamala:** As I sit at my computer today writing some of the last pages of *Suffering in Slow Motion*, I am filled with many emotions. I pray that the book will be a comfort to you, the one who reads it. I have tried to share my heart through words written on paper. It is not easy to get words off pages and into hearts, but I pray I have achieved this. In doing this, our family's suffering will have done some good, and for that we can be thankful.

The journey our family has been on for the past five years has been full of unpredictable changes and progressive suffering. It remains a mystery to us why we have been in this place for so long. Sometimes we wonder, why so long? For what possible good? Nevertheless, we are here, and although at times we feel we cannot make it through one more moment, we do. How? We have help.

First, we have a strong reliance on God and His sustaining presence in our lives. Second, we are determined to go through this in the best way we can, without regret. Last, we have the support of family and friends who have helped carry the load. God will always do His part when we ask Him for help—I know that for sure. Like the wind, I cannot see Him, but I feel Him and see what His presence can do.

If you are suffering from an illness or are the caregiver of someone who is, you can go your journey *alone* if you choose. But in the end, *alone* is not good. Your own strength will eventually be gone, and devoted family and friends can only go so far with you. For this reason I urge you to invite God to join you. When He comes into your life He will remain with you to the end and through the end, embracing you, sustaining and loving you until you are through suffering and on the other side of it, where there is rest and peace for everyone.

## Epilogue
### (written at the time of publication)

**Pamala:** My heart hurts today. I have been faced today with yet another change in my life due to Richard's horrible illness. I had to sell our home. It was the home in which I thought our family would celebrate Christmas, Easter and birthdays for years to come. Richard and I planted trees in this yard in hopes that, one day, our grandkids would swing and play under them. I dreamed of telling them stories of how Poppy Richard and I had planted these trees for them to enjoy when we first moved from California to Oklahoma. That was the plan; however it has not worked out that way. Instead I spent the day going through boxes in the attic, boxes that contained mine and Richard's life together, all neatly wrapped and put away for a while.

But reality has come to call, and I must face where the compass is pointing, accept the direction we are headed and move on. Richard and I have a wonderful past, but we will not have a future together. All the dreams we contemplated together as a couple have been altered greatly; the disease has changed everything.

I have faced this reality time and time again these past six years since his diagnoses, yet I face it once more today. This is part of the *suffering in slow motion* progression. You continue to bump into the reality of loss over and over again. The long good-bye is there every morning to greet you. You so yearn to be done with the dying if indeed there is no future, but you cannot, because the end is not yet. This is completely exhausting!

I was surprised, blindsided by my emotions today. I didn't see them coming at all. These surprise attacks come throughout a journey of suffering—days of tears and fears out of the blue, ambushing even the strongest of souls. It is all part of the process of letting go one inch at a time. You watch the suffering one still suffer, while trying your best to plan life, which will and must go on. The problem is my plan changes continuously.

My plan was to take care of Richard here in this house until he died. I had the contractor make changes in the original house plan to accommodate Richard's care in the future. I even spent over $35,000 just two years ago to provide for his needs more adequately as he became more debilitated. Still, in the end, no matter what I did to keep him here with me, I had to accept the fact that his particular needs could not be met here in this house. I had to let go of this plan, and figure out plan B.

Plan B necessitates me selling this very large home and moving to a much smaller one, a house that I will move into alone. Plan B will better suit our family's needs, as Richard's care is costly and I honestly do not need much room just for me. I say "just for me" because somewhere along the way our baby boy, Aaron, grew up and has left the nest. He recently got the opportunity to move back to California to live his dream of playing and singing in a professional band. He has been such a great help these past few years—what a trouper he has been for our family. He moved with us here to Oklahoma, leaving all of his friends when he was a sophomore in high school. It was not easy for him to adjust from the "California Surfer Joe" mentality to the dry flatland and slow pace of Oklahoma. Yet he did it with great grace. I know he will come back to visit, but the fact is, he is off and running toward his future, and I would not change that for anything.

When you sell a home you do more than just pack boxes and move furniture. You also leave tons of memories, etchings on your heart of moments spent there, echoes of "laughter in the hall"—in my case, sounds that will never be heard again. As I went through the attic boxes, I felt as if I was reliving the past twenty-seven years of my life. The boxes were filled with the typical stuff you pack away in the attic: the kids' toys, baby clothes, kindergarten pictures, handmade Mother's Day cards, sports trophies and family portraits with people sporting strange hairstyles. But also among the mishmash lay Richard's many tangible accomplishments, like boxes of his sermons on tape, files of future sermon ideas, projected budgets for church and school, wedding scripts, conference notes along with unending stacks of printed material he had written and distributed over the years. There were all the awards he had received, beginning in college and going all the way through the farewell party he was given when we left California. There were also books from his personal library, which he treasured. All had to be gone through, and I had to decide what to keep and what to give away.

I admit I sobbed my way through each and every box of memories. These were the tangible things I could touch, but they represented so much more. Every sermon he preached influenced lives; the weddings he conducted evolved into families; the students he taught now teach others; and for each goal accomplished, I was there to give a party and celebrate with him.

My life is filled with memories but life is in the doing, the living day to day, and because of the living and doing memories exist. It is life we must live for, not memories. Life pushes us forward while memories remind us of life lessons as well as treasured moments to savor. I do enjoy a walk down memory lane now and then, but I have never been one to live in the past. Rather I have used my past to help me live better in the present and look forward to the future. My future, though filled with uncertainties, will provide new memories to go along with the old.

I have a new house waiting to be lived in, and with the living there will most assuredly come new etchings on my heart. Richard and I were blessed to give life to three wonderful, eternal souls named Apryl, Amy and Aaron. Because of their lives and the life God has in store for me, the walls of my new home will one day once again resound with late night talks, beautiful sunsets, lots of music and laughter mingled with a few tears now and then, the pitter-patter of little feet, and in good time, the sounds of life.

# Appendix

## How and Where to Get Help From Home

### Aging

Administration on Aging
200 Independence Avenue, S.W., Room 309
Washington, D.C. 20201
(202) 619-0724
www.aoa.dhhs.gov

Aging for Healthcare Research and Quality
2101 E. Jefferson Street, Suite 501
Rockville, MD 20852
(301) 594-1364
www.ahcpr.gov

Aging Network Services
4400 East-West Highway, Suite 907
Bethesda, MD 20814
(301) 657-4329
www.againgnets.com

Children of Aging Parents
1609 Woodbourne Road, Suite 302-A
Levittown, PA 19057
(215) 945-6900
www.careguide.net

### AIDS

American Red Cross AIDS-Education Office
431 18th Street NW
Washington, D.C. 20006

(202) 639.3520
www.redcross.org/services/hss/hivaids
JAMA HIV/AIDS Information Center
www.amaassn.org/special/hiv/hivhome.htm

AIDS Education Global Information System
HIV/AIDS Information on the Internet
www.aegis.com

**ALS** (Amyotrophic Lateral Sclerosis)—Lou Gehrig's Disease
ALS Association
27001 Agoura Road, Suite 150
Calabasas Hills, CA 91301
(818) 880-9007
www.alsa.org

ALS Survival Guide
www.lougehrigsdisease.net

**Alcoholism**
National Institute on Alcohol Abuse & Alcoholism
600 Executive Boulevard, Willco Building
Bethesda, MD 20892-7003
www.niaaa.nih.gov

Alcoholics Anonymous
www.alcoholics-anonymous.org

Al-Anon/Alateen
www.al-anon.alateen.org

## Alzheimer's Disease

Alzheimer's Association
919 N. Michigan Avenue, Suite 1100
Chicago, IL 60611-1676
(800) 272-3900
www.alz.org

John Douglas French Foundation for Alzheimer's Disease
11620 Wilshire Boulevard
Los Angeles, CA 90025
(213) 470-5462
www.jdfaf.org

Alzheimer's Disease Education and Referral Center
P.O. Box 8250
Silver Springs, MD 20907-8250
(301) 495-3331 or (800) 438-4380
www.alzheimers.org

## Autism

Autism Society of America
7910 Woodmont Avenue, Suite 300
Bethesda, MD 20814-3067
(301) 657-0881 or (800) 3 AUTISM
www.autism-society.org

## Cancer

American Cancer Society
1599 Clifton Road, N.E.
Atlanta, GA 30329
(800) ACS-2345
www.cancer.org

American Institute for Cancer Research
1759 R Street N.W.
Washington, D.C. 20009
(202) 328-7744 or (800) 843-8114
www.aicr.org

National Cancer Institute
6116 Executive Boulevard, Suite 3036A
Bethesda, MD 20892-8322
(800) 4CANCER
www.cancer.gov

## Cardiology

American Heart Association
7272 Greenville Avenue
Dallas, TX 75231
(800) 242-8721
www.americanheart.org

American Medical Association Division of Cardiology
515 N. State Street
Chicago, IL 60610
(312) 464-500
www.ama-assn.org

## Crohn's Disease

Crohn's and Colitis Foundation of America
386 Park Avenue South, 17th Floor
New York, NY 10016
(212) 685-3440 or (800) 932-2423
www.ccfa.org

## Cystic Fibrosis

Cystic Fibrosis Foundation
6931 Arlington Road, Suite 200
Bethesda, MD 20814
(301) 951-4422 or (800) 344-4823
www.cff.org

Boomer Esiason Foundation
452 Fifth Avenue, Tower 22
New York, NY 10018
(212) 525-7777
www.esiason.org

Cystic Fibrosis Information on the Internet
www.cysticfibrosis.com

## Depression

Depression and Bipolar Support Alliance
730 N. Franklin Street, Suite 501
Chicago, IL 60610-7240
(312) 642-0049 or (800) 826-3632
www.dballiance.org

Copewithlife.com
7617 Mineral Point Road, Suite 300
Madison, MI 53717
(608) 827-2497 or (877) 272-3393
www.copewithlife.com

Dealing with Depression
www.depress.com

## Diabetes

American Diabetes Association
1701 North Beauregard Street
Alexandria, VA 22311
(703) 549-1500 or (800) DIABETES
www.diabetes.org

Diabetes Public Health Resource
CDC Division of Diabetes Translation
P.O. Box 8728
Silver Springs, MD 20910
(877) 232-3422
www.cdc.gov/diabetes

Juvenile Diabetes Research Foundation International
120 Wall Street, 19th Floor
New York, NY 10005-4001
(212) 785-9500 or (800) 533-2873
www.jdrf.org

## Down Syndrome

National Down Syndrome Society
666 Broadway
New York, NY 10012
(212) 460-9330 or (800) 221-4602
www.ndss.org

## Family Caregivers

Family Caregiver Alliance
690 Market Street, Suite 600
San Francisco, CA 94104
(415) 434-3388
www.caregiver.org

National Family Caregiver Association
10400 Connecticut Avenue, #500
Kensington, MD 20895-3944
(800) 896-3650
www.nfcacares.org

FamilyCare America
www.familycareamerica.com

## Huntington's Disease
Huntington's Disease Society of America
158 West 29th Street, 7th Floor
New York, NY 10001-5300
(800) 345-HDSA
www.hdsa.org

## Lupus
Lupus Foundation of America, Inc.
1300 Piccard Drive, Suite 200
Rockville, MD 20850-4303
(301) 670-9292 or (800) 558-0121
www.lupus.org

## Mental Health
National Mental Health Association
2001 N. Beauregard Street, 12th Floor
Alexandria, VA 22311
(703) 684-7722 or (800) 969-NMHA
www.nmha.org

National Institute of Mental Health
5600 Fishers Lane, Room 15C-05
Rockville, MD 20857
(301) 443-4513
www.nimh.nih.gov

Internet Mental Health
www.mentalhealth.com

**Multiple Sclerosis**
National MS Society
733 Third Avenue
New York, NY 10017
(212) 986-3240 or (800) FIGHTMS
www.nmss.org

MS Foundation
6350 North Andrews Avenue
Fort Lauderdale, FL 33309-2130
(954) 776-6805 or (800) 225-6495
www.msfacts.org

MS Association of America
706 Haddonfield Road
Cherry Hill, NJ 08002
(856) 488-4500 or (800) 532-7667
www.msaa.com

## Parkinson's Disease

The American Parkinson's Disease Association, Inc.
1250 Hylan Boulevard, Suite 4B
Staten Island, NY 10305
(718) 981-8001 or (800) 223-2732
www.apdaparkinson.com

The Parkinson's Disease Foundation
710 West 168th Street
New York, NY 10032-9982
(212) 923-4700 or (800) 923-4700
www.pdf.org

The National Parkinson Foundation, Inc.
1501 Ninth Avenue/Bob Hope Road
Miami, FL 33136
(305) 547-6666 or (800) 327-4545
www.parkinson.org

## Rheumatoid Arthritis

The Arthritis Foundation
1330 West Peachtree Street
Atlanta, GA 30309
(404) 872-7100 or (800) 283-7800
www.arthritis.org

## Sickle-Cell Anemia

Sickle Cell Disease Association of America
(310) 216-6363 or (800) 421-8453
www.sicklecelldisease.org

American Sickle Cell Anemia Association
10300 Carnegie Avenue
Cleveland Clinic East Office Building
Cleveland, OH 44106
(216) 229-8600
www.ascaa.org

## Spina Bifida

Spina Bifida Association of America
4590 MacArthur Boulevard N.W., Suite 250
Washington, D.C. 20007-4226
(800) 621-3141
www.sbaa.org

## Stroke

National Stroke Association
9707 East Easter Lane
Englewood, CO 80112
(303) 649-9299 or (800) STROKES
www.stroke.org

American Stroke Association
7272 Greenville Avenue
Dallas, TX 75231
(888) 4 STROKE
www.strokeassociation.org

## General Health Websites

www.webMD.com
www.healthlinkusa.com
www.mayohealth.com
www.pdr.net
www.nccam.nih.gov
www.altmedicine.com

## Christian Websites for those who suffer

www.restministries.org
www.joniandfriends.org

# Notes

### Chapter One
### *Life in the Cocoon*

1. Sue Monk Kidd, *When The Heart Waits* (San Francisco: Harper & Row, 1990), 10.
2. Dan Webster, *The Real Deal* (Grand Rapids, Mich.: Authentic Leadership, Inc., 1998), 94.
3. Kidd, 40.
4. Kidd, 26.
5. Thomas Merton as quoted in Kidd, 37.
6. Kidd, 49.

### Chapter Two
### *What Will Become of Me?*

1. Phillip Yancey, *Where Is God When It Hurts?* (Grand Rapids, Mich.: Zondervan, 1990), 184.
2. Yancey, 185.

### Chapter Three
### *What Is Suffering?*

1. Gerald L. Sittser, *A Grace Disguised: How the Souls Grows Through Loss* (Grand Rapids, Mich.: Zondervan, 1996), 56.
2. "The Good News About Depression" 1998 NetHealth, a division of Epicenter Communications, Inc. Available online at www.depression.com.
3. Michael Youssef, *If God is in Control Why is My Life Such a Mess?* (Nashville, Tenn.: Thomas Nelson, 1998), 19.

### Chapter Four
### *Trading Fear for Trust*

1. *Our Daily Bread*, February 20, 2002.
2. Archibald D. Hart, *The Anxiety Cure* (Nashville, Tenn.: Word, 1989), 27.

## Chapter Five
### *Keys to Living With Loss*

1. Roger Nix, "What To Do When Life Seems Diminished," Believer's Church, Tulsa, OK (January 11, 2002).
2. Rabbi David Wolpe, *Making Loss Matter* (New York: Riverhead Books, 1999), 129.
3. Viktor E. Frankl, *Man's Search for Meaning*, 4th edition (Boston: Beacon Press, 1992), 75.
4. Frankl, 78.
5. Frankl, 87.


## Chapter Six
### *When God* Doesn't

1. Rick Bragg, "Killer Wind Shakes Town." This article appeared in the *Modesto Bee* on April 3, 1994. Used by permission of the Associated Press.
2. Steven Lawson, *When All Hell Breaks Loose* (Colorado Springs: NavPress, 1993), 11.
3. Lawson, 14.
4. As quoted in Philip Yancey, *Where is God When It Hurts?*, 77.
5. James Dobson, *When God Doesn't Make Sense* (Wheaton, Ill.: Tyndale House Publishers, 1993), 41.
6. Harold S. Kushner, *When Bad Things Happen to Good People* (New York: Avon Books, 1981), 26.
7. Kushner, 33.
8. Kushner, 43.
9. Yancey, 96.


## Chapter Seven
### *Staying Close*

1. As quoted in Philip Yancey, *Where Is God When it Hurts?*, 168.


## Chapter Eight
### *The God of All Comfort*

1. Robert Heffler, *Will Daylight Come?* (Lima, Ohio: CSS Publishing

Company, 1979), 25-26. Used by permission from CSS Publishing Company, 517 S. Main Street, P.O. Box 4503, Lima, Ohio 45802-4503.

## Chapter Nine
### *The Importance of Family and Friends*

1. Steven J. Lawson, *When All Hell Breaks Loose* (Colorado Springs: NavPress, 1993), 71.

## Chapter Ten
### *Making the Hard Decisions*

1. Family Caregiver Alliance Fact Sheet: Selected Caregiver Statistics. Available online at www.caregiver.org.
2. Family Caregiver Alliance Fact Sheet.
3. Family Caregiver Alliance Fact Sheet.
4. Family Caregiver Alliance Fact Sheet.
5. Family Caregiver Alliance Fact Sheet.
6. Family Caregiver Alliance: Caregivers at Risk. Available online at www.caregiver.org.
7. Family Caregiver Alliance: Caregivers at Risk.
8. Family Caregiver Alliance: Caregivers at Risk.
9. Family Caregiver Alliance: Caregivers at Risk.
10. Family Caregiver Alliance: Caregivers at Risk.
11. Archibald D. Hart, *Adrenaline and Stress* (Nashville, Tenn.: Word, 1995), 20.
12. Hart, *Adrenaline and Stress*, 69.
13. Pat Curry, Dealing With Finances After the Death of a Loved One. Available online at www.bankrate.com.

## Chapter Eleven
### *Prayer and Journaling: Seeking the Father's Heart*

1. Loren Cunningham, *Is That Really You, God?* (Grand Rapids, Mich.: Chosen Books, 1984), 157-58.
2. Ron Dunn, *Will God Heal Me?* (Sisters, Ore.: Multnomah Books, 1997), 20.

Chapter Twelve
*The Long View: Keeping Your Eyes on the Horizon*

1.    Strong's Greek/Hebrew Definitions from PC Study Bible software
      program.